D1233906

RETHINKING
REPROGENETICS

Rethinking Reprogenetics

*Enhancing Ethical Analyses
of Reprogenetic Technologies*

Inmaculada de Melo-Martín

OXFORD
UNIVERSITY PRESS

OXFORD
UNIVERSITY PRESS

Oxford University Press is a department of the University of Oxford. It furthers
the University's objective of excellence in research, scholarship, and education
by publishing worldwide. Oxford is a registered trade mark of Oxford University
Press in the UK and certain other countries.

Published in the United States of America by Oxford University Press
198 Madison Avenue, New York, NY 10016, United States of America.

Library of Congress Cataloging-in-Publication Data
Names: de Melo-Martín, Inmaculada, author.
Title: Rethinking reprogenetics : enhancing ethical analyses of reprogenetic
technologies / by Inmaculada de Melo-Martín.
Description: Oxford ; New York : Oxford University Press, [2017] | Includes
bibliographical references.
Identifiers: LCCN 2016013522| ISBN 9780190460204 (hardcover : alk. paper) |
ISBN 9780190460228 (epub) | ISBN 9780190460211 (updf)
Subjects: | MESH: Reproductive Techniques, Assisted—ethics | Genetic
Enhancement—ethics
Classification: LCC RG133.5 | NLM WQ 208 | DDC 176/.2—dc23 LC record available
at http://lccn.loc.gov/2016013522

1 3 5 7 9 8 6 4 2

Printed by Sheridan Books, Inc., United States of America

For Cristina,

she is so much like her mom, her dad, and her brother

CONTENTS

ACKNOWLEDGMENTS

This book has benefited from the comments of friends and colleagues. Thanks are due to Stephen Brown, Ina Cholst, Sharon Crasnow, Malia Fullerton, Anita Ho, Kristen Intemann, Mary Mahowald, Laura Purdy, and Arleen Salles for their helpful suggestions and criticisms.

Much of this work was done during my 2015 sabbatical leave. I am thankful to Weill Cornell Medical College for sabbatical funding and to my Division Chief, Joseph Fins, for his support. Thanks also to Zev Rosenwaks and Ron MacKenzie for their continuing support of my work. Part of my sabbatical leave was spent at the University of Washington. I am grateful to the UW Philosophy Department for inviting me to be the *Benjamin Rabinowitz Visiting Professor in Medical Ethics*. It was while I was there that this project took final shape. I am particularly grateful to Sara Goering, Michael Rosenthal, and Alison Wylie for all their help during my stay. Thanks are also due to the students in my class, *Ethical Issues in Reproductive and Genetic Technologies*. Our discussions helped me clarify many of the arguments that appear in this book.

I am similarly indebted to Stephen Brown for pushing me to write this book and for offering me the space—literally and figuratively—to write a significant part of it. Thanks also to Lucy Randall, my editor at OUP, for her encouragement and support through all the stages of this project.

As always, I am grateful to and for my family and friends. They provide the love, support, wine-tasting trips, laughs, interesting conversations, and encouragement that make my work enjoyable, and their presence—even when they are absent—reminds me how lucky I am. Thanks to my nephew Martin and my niece Cristina for highlighting the value of what is unchosen.

Chapter 3 draws on "Sex Selection and the Procreative Liberty Framework," which appeared in 2013 in the *Kennedy Institute Ethics Journal* 23 (1):1–18. Thanks to the Johns Hopkins University Press for permission to use this material.

Chapter 1

Introduction

Challenging Mainstream Defenses of Reprogenetic Technologies

Molly Nash suffered from Fanconi anemia, a rare genetic disease (Belkin 2001). Without a bone marrow transplant, she would die before the age of 10, and a suitable donor was proving difficult to find. Molly's parents decided to undergo in vitro fertilization (IVF) and preimplantation genetic diagnosis (PGD) in order to select an embryo that would become a donor for Molly. These are the circumstances in which Adam Nash was born in August 2000. In 2008, researchers reported the birth of the first baby born after his mother, a carrier of an inherited mutation for early-onset hereditary breast cancer, had undergone IVF with PGD to select an embryo free of the genetic mutation in question (Jasper, Liebelt, and Hussey 2008). In December 2009, the direct-to-consumer genetic testing company, 23andMe, filed a patent that it claims will allow prospective parents to select gamete donors so as to have babies with chosen phenotypic characteristics including height, eye color, sex, and a variety of personality characteristics (DeFrancesco 2014). In October 2015, the United Kingdom legalized the use of mitochondrial replacement, a procedure that could allow women at risk of transmitting a mitochondrial disease to have unaffected children. Children born through these technologies will have DNA content from three different individuals rather than the usual two. These are but some of the ways in which reprogenetic technologies are now being used and could be used in the future. Why should we care about reprogenetic technologies? To be sure, these technologies, which combine the power of reproductive technologies with the tools of genetic science, are fascinating in many ways. They can provide newsworthy story lines about "three-parent babies" (Tingley, 2014) and offer suggestive scenarios for movies and novels (Huxley, [1932] 1998; Niccol 1997). But the current use of these technologies is relatively limited. In general, they are used by those suffering fertility problems or by those at a high risk of transmitting specific genetic mutations to their offspring. They are expensive and, in many cases, accessible only to those with the ability to pay for them out of their own pocket. The latest figures for the United States indicate that about 1.5% of all infants are conceived with the use of reproductive technologies such as IVF (CDC, American Society for Reproductive Medicine, and Society for Assisted Reproductive Technology 2014). In some European countries, the percentage of births assisted by reproductive technologies is higher: in Denmark in 2010, almost 6% of children were born with the help of these technologies, and in Slovenia more than 5% of them were so conceived (Kupka et al. 2014). Overall, however, the rates are relatively low. Similarly, whereas the use of reprogenetic technologies to create and screen embryos for a variety of mutations related to disease or disability or to select embryos of a preferred sex is now relatively routine, their use to create "perfect babies," or to enhance certain characteristics such as intelligence, strength, beauty, longevity, or self-control, is at present speculative.

It is true that many possible uses of reprogenetics are merely theoretical and that those that are not have a limited impact at present. But it would be a mistake to dismiss these technologies or to overlook the importance they might have for society simply because of their current, relatively marginal, role. Reprogenetic technologies affect some of the most important aspects of human existence: our desire to reproduce, to form families, to ensure the health and well-being of our offspring. They potentially give us an unprecedented and sophisticated level of control, not just over whether and when we wish to have children but also over what children we want to have, over who can and cannot be born. Indeed, some have argued that these technologies will allow us to transcend all human limitations so as to transform the human species into a different one of transhumans (Bostrom 2003). These advances thus present us with important ethical challenges. Even if one sets aside concerns about the possible use of reprogenetic technologies to radically overhaul our species, there are good reasons to believe that they can have profound effects on women, people with disabilities, and society in general. It is hardly surprising that they have received a significant amount of attention from the public, the general media, national and international policy-making bodies, and scholars from a variety of disciplines.

Mainstream proponents of reprogenetics believe that the transformative effects of these technologies, both current and future, are positive and should be welcomed. They argue that they increase reproductive choice, contribute to a reduction of suffering by eliminating genetic diseases and disabilities, and offer the opportunity to improve the human condition. Many also embrace these technologies for their potential ability to create beings who will have longer and healthier lives, better intellectual capacities, and more refined emotional experiences. Indeed, proponents often deem these technologies to be of such significance to human well-being that they take the raising of any concerns about reprogenetics as an obstacle to human progress. Some of the most vocal supporters, such as John Harris and Julian Savulescu, contend that the implementation of these technologies to select and enhance our offspring is such a benefit to humankind that it is not only morally permissible but morally required.

It is often difficult to decide how to respond to such enthusiastic and, as I will argue, usually simplistic appraisals of these technological interventions. When technologies affect central aspects of human existence such as reproduction and health, attempting to temper the fervor by calling attention to the various concerns that the technologies raise risks accusations of irrationality, obstructionism, Luddism, social conservatism, religious zealotry, and the like. Witness, for instance, the debate over the use of reprogenetic technologies to select embryos of the desired sex. Critics of this practice are accused not only of illegitimately interfering with peoples' reproductive liberties but also of being mystical, incoherent, and irrational (Harris 2005). Unsurprisingly, those who are less sanguine about these biomedical technologies are forced to be on the defensive, often feeling the need to preface their less enthusiastic—or completely disapproving—views by assuring the audience that they are not against scientific and technological development.

To be sure, some criticisms of reprogenetic technologies are grounded on misguided assumptions and questionable values. Nonetheless, at least some of them result not from irrationality or a desire to obstruct scientific and technological progress but from a view of science and technology that is more complex and arguably more sophisticated (Habermas 2003) than the one often found in the arguments of those enthusiastically defending reprogenetic technologies. Critics that conceive of scientific and technological advances as value-laden; shaped by social, ethical, and political values; influencing the way we see the world; and co-shaping some of the values that we hold dear are hardly irrational, irrelevant, or downright foolish, no matter how little one might agree with their conclusions. Consider, for example, the much-debated use of disgust as an appropriate moral guide in the assessment of reprogenetic technologies (Caplan 2003; Kaebnick 2008; Kass 1997; Midgley 2000; Niemelä 2011; Roache and Clarke 2009). Proponents of reprogenetics usually consider expressions of disgust to be irrational and use this as grounds for dismissing the concerns conveyed by this emotional response (Harris 1998, 2007). But although the use[1] of disgust as a reliable moral indicator can be questioned, it does not follow that the concerns expressed by such an emotion are all inconsequential or that such an emotional response is wholly irrational (Salles and de Melo-Martin 2012). Some studies suggest, for example, that these indistinct appeals to a sense of moral repugnance voice a need to recognize the uncertainty involved in risk evaluations of new technologies and the possible limitations of even the best studies (Wynne 2001, 2006). At least some expressions of repugnance can then be interpreted as communicating concerns about a lack of intellectual humility and institutional accountability on the part of scientists and policymakers. They thus express a value judgment about the quality of scientific and political institutions that fail to publicly discuss issues of responsibility for the inherent limitations of the knowledge they produce and defend. One might certainly disagree with these concerns, but to dismiss them as simply irrational, the result of religious zealotry, suggests a skewed understanding of rationality.

Moreover, many of the presuppositions underlying the technological imperative that guides much eager embracement of reprogenetics are not any less problematic or faulty than those of some opponents of reprogenetic technologies. Indeed, claims that a critical approach to science and technology is necessarily obstructionist, perverse, and mistaken simply misconceive both the role of science and technology in society and human existence and the role of ethical assessments of scientific and technological advances. Science and technology transform human beings as well as societies in profound and significant ways. One need not attach negative valance to technologies to adopt a critical stance toward reprogenetics. Although this is how proponents of reprogenetics often frame the debate, the contrast is not between understanding science and technology as positive on the one hand and conceiving of it as negative on the other, nor between progressive values and conservative ones. Neither is it a conflict between seeing science and technology as inseparable from our humanity or regarding such practices as artificial or unnatural. The contrast is—or so I will argue—between conceptualizing science and technology as value-neutral, thus framing technological innovations as mere tools for the improvement of humans and society, and conceiving of them as value-laden, as co-shaping human beings and the societies we develop. Insofar as science and technology are value-laden in a variety of ways, a critical stance toward these practices need not entail their rejection. It can involve an interest in reflecting on the kinds of societies we think better allow human beings to flourish and in using this as a guide to decide what kinds of scientific and technological developments we should embrace.

The purpose of this book is to challenge the enthusiastic acceptance of reprogenetics. Its task is hence primarily a critical one. My goal is to examine the arguments that have been offered to support the use of these technologies for selection and enhancement of our offspring and to call attention to the problematic assumptions that ground such defenses. This work engages and contests the positions of some of the main supporters of reprogenetics, including Nicholas Agar, Allen Buchanan, Nick Bostrom, David DeGrazia, Ronald Green, John Harris, John Robertson, Julian Savulescu, and Lee Silver. Although the arguments of these authors vary in scope and tone, all of them have ardently defended the development and implementation of reprogenetic technologies to select and enhance human offspring, and their arguments are examined throughout the book. Because of their prominent position in the debate, the attention that they have given to reprogenetic technologies in their work, the radical nature of many of their theses, and their cheerleading attitude toward these technologies, I will focus particularly on the works of Harris and Savulescu.

As the examples given earlier show, reprogenetic technologies can be used to select for genetic mutations or variants associated with diseases and disabilities. In the future, these technologies might be used to manipulate such genetic mutations in embryos or gametes in order to create unaffected children. Although the use of these technologies for these purposes is widely accepted, serious concerns exist about it. Many have called attention to the problematic assumptions about the value of a life with disabilities that underlie the defense of these technologies and to the negative consequences for people thought to be disabled, as well as society in general, that might follow from their use (see, for instance, Asch 1999, 2003; Barnes 2014; Garland-Thomson 2012; Goering 2008; Mills 2011; Parens and Asch 1999; Scully 2008; Shakespeare 2006; Wasserman and Asch 2006, 2014). More controversial still is the utilization of reprogenetics to select or modify genetic variations that are unrelated to disease, such as sex, hair or skin color, height, or beauty. Currently, these technologies can be used to select for or against one of these traits: sex. In the future, scientific and technological advances might allow prospective parents to select or manipulate at least some others.

Of course, I recognize that what counts as a disease or non-disease trait or characteristic is not clear cut. One has only to remember the fact that homosexuality was considered a psychiatric disorder until the early 1970s to realize this. Indeed, the concept of disease itself is a contested one (e.g., Boorse 1975; Reznek 1987). Nonetheless, reasonable arguments can be offered that at least some traits, such as hair or eye color, female or male sex, or particular degrees of strength, are appropriately thought to not involve disease—even when variations in such traits (e.g., short stature) might be "treated" by the medical profession. In assessing supporters' defenses, I focus primarily on this aspect of reprogenetics. Of course, the problematic assumptions that I discuss here affect both disease-related and non–disease-related uses of these technologies. Nonetheless, some questionable assumptions regarding what constitutes a disability or its effects on quality of life that ground mainstream defenses of reprogenetics are not directly addressed in this book, although related concerns will be considered.

The Approach

The analysis presented here has three characteristics currently missing from mainstream defenses of reprogenetic technologies. First, it is performed from a philosophical perspective that appreciates scientific and technological knowledge and practices as well as the uncertainties, ambiguities, and ignorance that accompanies their development and implementation. It seems clear that good ethics—and good public policy—regarding scientific and technological advances requires knowledge of such advances. If one wants to make claims about what follows ethically from particular biotechnological developments, one must be familiar with biomedical science and technology. For instance, we must know something about how genes work and what genetic testing techniques do in order to propose the existence of an obligation to obtain genetic information about our offspring or to ponder whether justice requires that we allow people to enhance genetic traits. Similarly, it would clearly be unhelpful to staunchly defend prospective parents' right to select the sex of their offspring if we lacked the scientific knowledge or technological ability to do so.

This attention to existing scientific and technological knowledge is particularly important in the debate over reprogenetics, in which it is often difficult to distinguish between what is currently possible, what available evidence suggests may at some point be possible, and what is complete fiction. For instance, when discussing genetic enhancement, proponents of reprogenetic technologies make few distinctions between our likely ability to manipulate human traits that are influenced by single genes, such as some diseases (e.g., Tay-Sachs, Huntington's disease), and our capacity to tinker with other, more complex and multifactorial diseases that involve the influence of multiple genes at multiple sites, epigenetic effects, and environmental factors among many other variables. This is an important caveat in a debate that frequently speaks of a future ability to enhance cognitive, character, and behavioral traits as if the genetic bases for these characteristics were as "simple" as those involved in single-gene traits. In Savulescu's own words:

> Intelligence, of many kinds: memory, temperament, patience, empathy, a sense of humour, optimism and just having a sunny temperament can profoundly affect our lives. All of these characteristics will have some biological and psychological basis capable of manipulation with technology (Savulescu 2005, 37).

No evidence exists that we will ever be able to genetically modify these traits in any significant way, and indeed, current scientific knowledge about human biology gives us reason to doubt such a possibility. This is the case not just because of the complexities of the traits but also because their characterization involves value judgments that have nothing to do with the biology. Take, for instance, a sense of humor. Anyone who has traveled to other countries and found herself puzzled by what makes the locals laugh is well aware that whatever the biological or genetic aspects that influence people's sense of humor, this complex trait involves multifaceted social and cultural interactions and norms, value judgments, and language processing and recognition features. And even if one is able to figure out the humor in a particular instance, the degree of emphasis a society places on humor is bound to affect the importance one gives to modifying such a trait.

But it is not just the issue of "ought," implying "can," that grounds the importance of having appropriate knowledge and understanding of relevant science and technology. Debating reprogenetic technologies in a context in which outlandish claims are made about what prospective parents will be able to do, does little to promote an informed public dialogue. Discussions of reprogenetics not uncommonly present as reality or as a likely possibility what is in fact just wishful thinking, from immortal beings, to intellects that can read books in seconds, to people immune to diseases. In democratic societies, it is essential that people be reliably informed about scientific advances. The public should know what current biomedical research can accomplish as well as what is improbable. Overconfidence in the power of science prevents a correct evaluation of the ethical and social implications of biomedical science and technology. It helps no one, and it certainly does not help democratic participation, to have the public and policymakers believing that genetic enhancement of our offspring, for instance, is a simple endeavor and a mere question of political will.

Of course, most proponents of reprogenetics are likely to include some note of caution when singing the praises of these technologies. But usually this is a mere formality that serves to introduce scientific research intended to buttress their optimistic claims, or it is essentially no more than a means of recognizing the technical difficulties involved in manipulating the particular traits under discussion while simultaneously assuring readers that the possibilities of doing so are not far away. In most cases, however, the discussions surrounding these technologies simply proceed as if scientific and technological limitations were a matter of no concern or did not exist at all.

Obviously, this does not mean that we should put off concerning ourselves with the ethical aspects of potential scientific and technological advances until they become reality. Such theoretical possibilities, which are legion when it comes to reprogenetic technologies, can serve as appropriate tools to inquire into the nature of human self-understanding, the scope of human rights, or the value of particular social practices. But in performing such analyses, scholars should ensure that they also offer a realistic evaluation of the feasibility of reprogenetic technologies for achieving such goals.

Mainstream discussions of reprogenetics rarely manage to maintain a responsible balance between contemplating theoretical possibilities that might emerge from current technological advances and offering a sober evaluation of their probability. As a result, engaging with proponents of reprogenetic technologies can prove tricky if one is inclined to take scientific and technological knowledge seriously. Their use of the scientific evidence is often problematic. Advocates of reprogenetic technologies not uncommonly present empirical evidence as a matter of scientific consensus when in fact it is highly contested (DeGrazia 2013; Persson and Savulescu 2008). Moreover, they often overinterpret the available data to arrive at unjustified conclusions about what these technologies can or will accomplish (DeGrazia 2013; Persson and Savulescu 2008; Savulescu 2005). As a result, critics find themselves obliged to point out that much of the discussion about what prospective parents will be able to do is scientifically and technological implausible while at the same time addressing the ethical issues raised by the unrealistic science. In most of this work, I endeavor to do exactly that: call attention to fanciful expectations while accepting reprogenetic proponents' examples at face value in order to assess the ethical arguments they make.

This concern with speculation extends not only to discussions about what we might or might not be able to know and do with reprogenetic technologies but also to the evaluation of the associated risks and potential benefits. As we shall see, proponents of reprogenetics extoll the prospective benefits of these technologies while downplaying the risks and dismissing concerns about uncertainty and caution. Ironically, supporters often contend that to talk about very serious risks to individuals or society is an exercise in speculation and warn against blocking the development of technologies with great potential simply because of what they deem to be conjectures. That the potential benefits such technologies could provide are just as speculative—if not more so—does not seem a cause for concern. On the one hand, they dismiss the possibility that these technologies might contribute to sexist practices, increase injustice, or negatively affect the health of future generations; on the other, they are perfectly happy to cite as potential benefits the prospect that future generations will not have to deal with a variety of diseases and disabilities, that the technologies could eventually become accessible to most people, and that, rather than reinforcing sexism, they could even contribute to improving the status of women.

In spite of proponents' disregard for these issues, concerns about uncertainties, about whether there is or can be enough reliable knowledge regarding certain aspects of these technologies (e.g., what the effects of germline modifications might be), or about what we should do when facing inevitable ignorance (i.e., march ahead or cautiously hold back) are also of crucial importance (Jonas 1984; Wynne 2001). Given the qualitative difference introduced by reprogenetics technologies, to disregard concerns about uncertainty and ignorance is highly problematic. This is an important epistemological issue that has moral significance. One can agree that some evaluations of risks and potential benefits are as good as they can currently be while still contending that such evaluations do not go far enough. Indeed the language of risks obscures the fact that much is unknown about the effects of using these technologies. Attention to uncertainties regarding long-term consequences, to unanticipated effects of the development and implementation of reprogenetics is necessary for an appropriate evaluation of these technologies. Nonetheless, proponents' discussions about the reliability of evaluations of risks and benefits often fail to recognize the limits of the knowledge that they advance.

Worries about uncertainty, speculation, and unrealistic expectations are not only a scientific issue but also an ethical one (de Melo-Martin 2010). It is ethically problematic to systematically evade discussions about the possibility that even the best scientific data (and in the case of reprogenetic technologies, such data are decidedly scarce) and the best assessments may be limited. If such considerations are excluded from the debate, it is unlikely that institutional regulations and safety mechanisms will be developed to deal with such unknown consequences. This is not an irrational demand intended to eliminate uncertainty for scientific and technological applications or to require that no risks be present. It is a call to seriously deliberate about the goals that we want to achieve with particular innovations and about appropriate or inappropriate trust in social institutions to deal with the unexpected impacts of these technologies. One can accept uncertainties when the ends pursued are thought to be worthwhile and there is trust that the institutional response to the uncertainties will be an adequate one. But such uncertainties can be reasonably rejected when the goals are unclear or of dubious value, when they are deemed to be important but not urgent, or when the trustworthiness of institutional responses is unclear.

Given these considerations, it is important to pay attention both to what we know and to what we do not know: what science tells us, what technology allows us to do, and the uncertainties that inevitably attach to scientific and technological knowledge and implementation. This is not simply because attending to such considerations is likely to provide a better account of reprogenetics but also because it can provide us with insights on how to better deal with risks, take fuller advantage of potential benefits, and manage unexpected consequences. The present analysis thus challenges mainstream evaluations of reprogenetics for failing to take into account current scientific knowledge and failing to strike a balance between theoretical speculation and assessment of what might come to be.

A feminist perspective is the second characteristic of my analysis that is absent from the work of the enthusiastic reprogenetics supporters discussed here. This perspective is most obvious in my use of gender as an analytical category that can help expose the important ways in which gender organizes and influences the development and implementation of reprogenetic technologies. As feminist scholars have amply shown, because of historical systems of oppression, gender (as well as race, class, sexual orientation, and other social categories) has influenced the world and structured the social and material circumstances and experiences of individuals in particular ways. People's social location (i.e., their gender, race, ethnicity, and class) shapes their social roles, their power, the norms to which they are subject, and their subjective identities. These social categories affect people's understanding of the world, shape the production of knowledge, and influence relationships with others. Feminists have therefore advocated the importance of attending to the ways in which these social categories in general, and gender in particular, organize and influence scientific, technological, and social phenomena. In taking gender as an analytical category, the present work is able to reveal both the striking absence of any significant discussion about women's roles in the works of mainstream supporters of reprogenetics and also the relevance of women's contributions to the development and use of these technologies, the unequal burdens that affect them, and the differential impacts that these technologies have on women's bodies and lives.

To use gender as a category of analysis when evaluating reprogenetics need not presuppose an essentialist view of women. There is little doubt that reprogenetic technologies affect differently situated women in varied ways. White, economically well-off women are the typical users of reprogenetics (Spar 2006), and they are encouraged to use these technologies to conceive genetically related children. On the other hand, poor women are often the ones providing eggs and serving as gestational carriers (Dickenson 2011; Donchin 2010; Twine 2015). Likewise, women who are thought to be at higher risk of having children considered disabled are encouraged to use these technologies to avoid bringing into the world children with particular diseases and disabilities (Parens and Asch 1999; Scully 2008; Shakespeare 2006; Tremain 2001). Divergences among differently situated women notwithstanding, commonalities also exist and are relevant. Use of gender as a category of analysis does not deny that the intersectionality of gender with other social categories (e.g., race, disability status, class, nationality) is likely to provide unique insights. However, this does not mean that attention to gender is unhelpful in trying to provide tools that contribute to undermining structures of sexual oppression and injustice (Haslanger 2000).

Another result of the feminist perspective espoused here is the attention to the gendered nature of scientific and technological knowledge and practices. Feminist scholars have offered compelling arguments showing that scientific knowledge and technological innovations are far from gender-neutral (e.g., Anderson 2004; Haraway 1988; Harding 1986; Keller 1985; Longino 1987; Mahowald 2000; Rolin 2004; Wajcman 2004; Wylie and Nelson 2007). Feminists have challenged the apparent gender-neutrality of our common notions of objectivity and scientific methodology (Code 1991; Haraway 1988; Harding 1991; Schiebinger 1989), have called attention to the gender biases inherent in past and present scientific theories (Fausto-Sterling 1992; Haraway 1989; Hrdy 1986; Jordan-Young 2010; Lloyd 2005; Spanier 1995), and have criticized the disregard in scientific and technological development for issues of concern to women and other marginalized groups (Harding 2008; Schiebinger 2004; Wajcman 2004). The authors discussed here, on the other hand, either neglect or deny the gendered nature of scientific and technological knowledge and practices. One of the tasks of this work is to show that in doing so they provide us with evaluations of reprogenetics that are inadequate. Moreover, because they ignore the gendered aspects of science and technology, they fail to challenge the ways in which some of those aspects promote knowledge, policies, and practices that disadvantage women, and they miss the opportunity to influence such knowledge, policies, and practices so as to reduce injustices against women.

The third distinctive aspect of the present analysis, which is inextricably related to the feminist perspective, is its insistence that the social and political context in which scientific and technological practices are developed and implemented must be taken into account to provide a meaningful evaluation of reprogenetics. Science and technology are not just gendered; they also shape and are shaped by the social structures within which they take place. They incorporate, promote, reinforce, and challenge particular values. By doing so, they influence, and are influenced by, the societies that we construct (Floridi and Sanders 2004; Idhe 1993; Jasanoff 2004; Latour 2005; Swierstra and Waelbers 2012; Verbeek 2005; Winner 1980). Technological developments change human actions and mediate the reasons we have to act. Technologies can allow and forbid, encourage and block, alter and reinforce human actions. They reveal reality in new ways, influencing the reasons and motivations that underpin our perception of what is real, fostering ideas about what we ought to do, and shaping our assessment of which options are practical. If this is so, then a decontextualized analysis of reprogenetics will fail to reveal the interactions between the technologies we develop and the societies we have, the ways in which science and technology mediate the relations between human beings and the world.

Of course, eliminating or minimizing contextual factors can be an appropriate heuristic approach in some cases. It can help us focus on a particular aspect of a scientific or technological development. Moreover, any evaluation of a given technological innovation will inevitably set aside at least some contextual factors simply because they are legion and it is difficult, if not impossible, to take them all into account. Choices must be made about which aspects are most salient, but dealing with reprogenetic technologies as if the social context were irrelevant is, I contend, mistaken. As with their neglect of gender, decontextualized evaluations of reprogenetics necessarily miss important features, are likely to contribute to injustice, and fail to challenge conditions of oppression.

The co-shaping of science, technology, and society is not alone in being neglected in mainstream analyses of reprogenetics. When the ethical implications of the development and implementation of reprogenetics are considered, the social context is also ignored or, at best, paid lip service. For instance, the typical justification for the development and implementation of reprogenetic technologies is that they increase women's reproductive freedom. But when appeals are made to women's reproductive liberty, it is important to examine the viable choices women have given the particular social context. The fact that these technologies allow women options that they might not have had before is insufficient to claim that they increase reproductive freedom. The social context in which women make their choices might not only constrain their ability to use these technologies (e.g., if they lack the financial means) but also exert pressure to use them (e.g., if they are likely to transmit particular diseases or disabilities to their children).

This disregard for the social context in which reprogenetics are developed and implemented is also obvious in the ways in which proponents of these technologies attempt to solve some of the problems that reprogenetics might create. For example, most of the authors discussed here contemplate the objection that the use of reprogenetic technologies to enhance particular traits (e.g., intelligence) could, in our current social context, exacerbate existing unjust inequalities because only those with ability to pay for the technologies will have access to them. One common response to this concern is to suggest that governments should make reprogenetics, or some of their uses, available to everyone (Harris 2007). Access to reprogenetics for everyone would, advocates believe, address the problem of increasing inequalities while simultaneously allowing prospective parents to use these technologies to improve their offspring's well-being. If we lived in a world in which limited resources were not a problem; in which the inability to have genetically related offspring was the most pressing concern; and in which the persistence of genetic diseases, the existence of unenhanced cognitive capacities, and the lack of control over the sex of one's offspring constituted the main causes of preventable death, suffering, and misery, such a solution would be quite appropriate. However, as should be obvious, if such a world exists, we do not inhabit it. In our world, children find themselves in desperate need of good homes, pregnant women lack the basic access to health care that would allow them to improve their own and their future children's well-being, and parents are unable to provide nutritious food to their children—all of which would go a long way to improve children's cognitive capacities. In our world, preventing most cases of premature death requires not advanced technological interventions but access to existing treatments such as vaccines for tuberculosis or to basic amounts of food, and what limits children's well-being is not unenhanced cognitive capacities, a lack of talent for music or sport, or shyness and impatience but the inability to obtain food, clean water, and education and to live in societies with social structures that allow them to thrive. Of course, all of these problems are not going to be solved simply by providing a contextualized evaluation of reprogenetics. However, the stance adopted when scrutinizing these technologies—in a utopian vacuum or in the current social and political context—has a considerable impact on how we evaluate them, what aspects of their development and use we emphasize, what impacts we take to be salient, and what solutions we offer.

The Challenge

Undoubtedly, any attempt to reflect on reprogenetic technologies requires some understanding of what these technologies involve, what they do, and how they are or can be used. To this end, chapter 2 of this book offers a brief description of reprogenetic technologies, which I understand here to mean the combination of reproductive technologies and genetic tools aimed at reproduction rather than simply at research. I pay particular attention to IVF and PGD, both because they are the "basic" tools in reprogenetics and because they are currently in widespread use. But I also discuss newer techniques that are receiving a significant amount of attention, including genome editing tools such as the CRISPR/Cas9 system and reproductive techniques such as mitochondrial replacement. As mentioned earlier, discussions of reprogenetics frequently fail to distinguish what we can currently do with these technologies from what we expect to be able to do with them in the future and from what appears to be complete fiction. Chapter 2 takes care to distinguish uses that have become routine in a clinical context from those, such as enhancement possibilities involving both somatic and germline modifications, that at this point are mostly speculative.

Reproductive and genetic technologies raise a variety of ethical challenges in and of themselves. However, when used separately or in combination, the goals they seek differ in morally relevant ways. As a stand-alone technology, IVF is typically used to help people with fertility problems conceive genetically related children.[1] Genetic technologies can be employed for at least three different purposes: to test for the presence of particular mutations or variants in an individual's genome via genetic testing or screening; to treat certain medical conditions influenced by specific genetic mutations by inserting normal genes into the genome of a person with a serious illness via gene transfer techniques; and to identify particular individuals, usually for legal reasons such as establishing paternity or implicating or excluding suspects in crime proceedings, via DNA fingerprinting.

When combined to form what is termed "reprogenetic technologies," the ends pursued via reproductive and genetic

---

1. IVF and associated technologies can also allow the conception of offspring to whom the prospective parents have no genetic connection (e.g., when both the oocytes and the sperm are donated), but these technologies are most commonly used to enable at least one of the partners to have a genetic connection to the future child.

technologies go beyond helping people reproduce and diagnosing and treating certain conditions. The main goals sought become the selection of embryos with or without particular genetic muta-tions or variants or the creation of embryos with specific genetic characteristics. The aim is to conceive offspring who have or lack specifically chosen traits. This is not to say that the ethical issues that reproductive, genetic, and reprogenetic technologies raise do not overlap at all; they certainly do. Reprogenetic technolo-gies are used by people who have fertility problems, by those at risk of passing on certain genetic mutations, and by those who are interested in having genetically related offspring. Hence, ethical issues concerning reproductive and genetic technologies can also be relevant to reprogenetics. Nonetheless, reprogenetic technologies present us with unique concerns. An overview of these technologies can help us better understand what those issues are.

Chapters 3 to 8 challenge mainstream defenses of repro-genetics as offered by well-known proponents such as Agar, Buchanan, Bostrom, DeGrazia, Green, Robertson, Silver, and particularly Harris and Savulescu. Chapters 3 and 4 directly address the main arguments given by several of these authors to defend the use of these technologies. Specifically, chapter 3 tackles arguments defending the moral permissibility of repro-genetic technologies grounded on procreative or reproductive liberty. Reproduction, not unreasonably, is seen by most people as central to an individual's identity and as an important fea-ture of one's life projects. For this reason, there is significant support for a presumption against interference with people's reproductive choices. It is thus not surprising that mainstream proponents of reprogenetics have used procreative freedom as the main argument to defend the development and use of these technologies. In chapter 3, however, I contest such an argu-ment. I maintain that appeals to procreative freedom do little to settle important questions about the permissibility of using reprogenetic technologies, particularly when the technologies are used to select or enhance genetic variants or traits that are usually thought to be unrelated to disease, such as sex, hair or skin color, height, or beauty. Proponents of reprogenetics have vociferously defended this use as falling under the scope of procreative liberty. In chapter 3, I first call attention to the lack of agreement on the existence, nature, and scope of reproductive liberty in general. I then contend that even if one accepts that procreative freedom entails the right *to* procreate, further argument is needed to show that such a right also encompasses a right to have a *particular* child, which is exactly what reprogenetic technologies aim to achieve. I then evaluate proponents' arguments purporting to prove that procreative freedom entails the liberty to use reprogenetic technologies to select or enhance one's offspring, and I show that they fail. I further argue that even if one were to agree that selection and enhancement fall within the scope of a right to reproduce, proponents' contention that no relevant harms can be proven to result from the use of reprogenetics is unpersuasive. I show that such is the case because they rely on problematic normative assumptions about what constitutes harm and how evidence of harm should be assessed. Because sex selection is currently not only possible but increasingly used by prospective parents and because it has been explicitly supported by proponents of reprogenetic technologies as clearly deserving of the strong protections associated with procreative liberty, my discussion focuses on sex selection. The arguments presented in chapter 3, however, can be applied to other non–disease-related traits.

Chapter 4 challenges arguments about a putative moral obligation to use reprogenetic technologies to select or enhance future offspring. Although many supporters of reprogenetics have contented themselves with defending the moral permissibility of these technologies, Harris and Savulescu have made the much bolder—and implausible—claim that the use of these technologies even to select for or enhance genetic traits unrelated to disease constitutes a moral duty. In chapter 4, I reject these claims on three different grounds. First, I argue that Savulescu and Harris fail to offer plausible justification for a moral obligation to select or enhance future children, and thus they provide no good reasons to believe that such obligations exist. I further show that should the existence of these obligations be granted, their usefulness in guiding the decisions and actions of prospective parents is dubious. Finally, I argue that even if these moral obligations could serve as guides to action, the negative consequences that are likely to follow from endorsing and fulfilling these putative moral duties call into question their acceptability.

After showing that the arguments offered to support the moral permissibility and obligatoriness of reprogenetic technologies to select and enhance non–disease-related traits fail, chapters 5 through 7 tackle three problematic assumptions that underpin mainstream appraisals of reprogenetics: that attempting to control the natural lottery with these technologies is advisable and possible and that the technologies themselves are both gender-neutral and value-neutral. These assumptions have different roles in the assessments of reprogenetics technologies presented by proponents. Their presuppositions about the degree of control over the natural lottery that these technologies could give us and about the desirability of exercising such control leads them to see these tools as more beneficial than is reasonable. Their assumptions about the gender- and value-neutrality of reprogenetics lead them to ignore a variety of considerations that, when taken into account, would lead, if not to a rejection, to a very different appraisal of the technologies.

In Chapter 5, I challenge proponents' claims about the degree of control that reprogenetic technologies are thought to afford prospective parents. Without denying that these technologies will permit a certain degree of power over which children are brought into the world, I reject proponents' ambitions of control over the natural lottery as unwise and illusory. By examining some advocates' own beliefs about the sorry state of affairs for which human beings are responsible, I question whether humans have the wisdom to appropriately control sexual reproduction and direct human evolution. More importantly, I show that proponents' exaggerated claims about the control that reprogenetic technologies will give us are grounded on an untenable genetic determinism. To be sure, advocates explicitly reject a deterministic view of human genetics. Nonetheless, I show in this chapter that without the assumption of genetic determinism, proponents' ambitions of control are unintelligible. Attending to the complexity of human biology in general, and of the traits that are the concern of proponents specifically, undermines genetic determinism and shows that human beings' ability to reliably control such traits is much more limited than they would have us believe.

Although all the authors discussed here are presumably aware that reprogenetic technologies have differential effects on men and women, their analysis betrays a blatant disregard for the implications of these differential effects. In chapter 6, I call attention to the absence of a gendered analysis of reprogenetic technologies and argue that gender-neutral evaluations are problematic for a variety of reasons. First, and most obviously, supporters offer a mistaken description of reprogenetics. Only women's bodies are directly implicated in the use and development of these technologies. Women are the ones who undergo IVF and who provide the eggs needed for both the development and the implementation of reprogenetics. Women gestate, give birth to, and usually rear the babies who are conceived, selected, and perhaps at some point enhanced with the help of such technologies. Moreover, all the genetic interventions necessary for selecting and enhancing embryos require the use of IVF and thus, again, the implication of women's bodies and their reproductive materials. Therefore, gender-neutral analyses of reprogenetics simply conceal the differential burdens that these technologies impose on men's and women's bodies. Second, gender-neutral evaluations also mask the unequal effects that reproductive decisions have on men's and women's lives which also overburden women. Although proponents of reprogenetics often use the rhetoric of choice to defend these technologies, their gender-neutral analysis betrays a disregard for the ways in which the presumed increase in choices can actually contribute to restricting the options of many individual women and can affect women's status. Finally, gender-neutral evaluations of reprogenetics are likely to further injustices against women. This is the case, I argue, because they disregard the ways in which the actual development and implementation of these technologies can contribute to overburdening women and because they implicitly and uncritically sanction a status quo that systematically disadvantages women.

Chapter 7 deals with another problematic assumption that grounds the defense of reprogenetic technologies presented by the authors under analysis: the value-neutrality of science and technology. In chapter 7, I discuss the thesis that science and technology are value-neutral or value-free and call it into question. I show that, although common, the belief in the value-neutrality of science and technology is nonetheless questionable for a variety of reasons. First, like a belief in the gender-neutrality of reprogenetic technologies, the value-free thesis presents an implausible view of scientific and technological practices that we would do well to abandon. Second, this belief has problematic implications for the assessment of science and technology. By taking ethical, social, and political values to be irrelevant, the assumption that scientific and technological developments are value-neutral limits the ethical evaluation of reprogenetic technologies to an assessment of risk and potential benefits and thus leads to a neglect of other relevant normative concerns. Additionally, the belief in the value-neutrality of science and technology renders democratic participation in scientific and technological policy-making unnecessary. To the extent that these activities are value-neutral, it would seem that the only pertinent factors in their evaluation are scientific and technical ones. Therefore, only the opinions of scientists and engineers, and not those of citizens in general, are essential to technology assessment, because only they have the relevant scientific and technical expertise.

Contrary to what proponents of reprogenetics assume, these technologies are not value-neutral or value-free. Ethical, social, and political values shape and are shaped by these technologies. Chapter 7 discusses some of the ways in which these technologies mediate, and thus create and transform, people's realities and reasons for action; how they affect the solutions that are taken as appropriate; how they challenge or reinforce particular values; and how they affect our ideas of what is right or wrong, virtuous or vicious, good or bad, morally obligatory or forbidden. Of course, the chapter does not present an exhaustive review of the multiple and diverse ways in which reprogenetics are value-laden. Its goal is simply to illustrate this fact so as to call attention to the problematic implications of the value-neutrality thesis.

Finally, chapter 8 offers an illustration of what a more adequate assessment of reprogenetic technologies—one that attends to context, is gendered, and recognizes the value-laden nature of these technologies—would look like. It focuses on mitochondrial replacement, a new technological development that allows the creation of an embryo with genetic material from three different people, two of whom are women. Unlike other reprogenetic technologies currently in use, mitochondrial transfer results in germline modifications and, as such, its effects on future generations are unknown. In chapter 8, I show that even if one were to accept that these techniques have a reasonable safety profile (and at this point that would be a very big assumption indeed), attention to the ends that these techniques will presumably help achieve and to the values that they reinforce and oppose calls for skepticism about their moral permissibility.

Why it Matters

In challenging the enthusiastic acceptance of reprogenetics, I want to go beyond insisting that the arguments offered by mainstream proponents of these technologies are flawed and unpersuasive, even though that is a crucial task of this book. The assumptions that ground much of the support for reprogenetics—assumptions, for example, about the role of technologies in improving human well-being; about what prospective parents owe their offspring; about how to create conditions for human flourishing; and about how to understand health, disease, and disability—have significant implications for how we want to proceed regarding these biomedical technologies. It is therefore important that we reflect on such assumptions carefully. But with this analysis I also aim to accomplish other goals. First, I want to resist, and call upon others to contest, the tendency in bioethics and in medicine to embrace technological innovations as mere tools that can be used appropriately or inappropriately and that call only for an assessment of the potential benefits and risks, usually narrowly understood, of such use. Not, of course, that conceptualizing technologies as mere tools is always inappropriate. Nonetheless, they are much more than that, and this complexity should be acknowledged and attended to.

Second, I also wish to reject the equally common propensity to accept technological fixes as the best, or even adequate, solutions to complicated aspects of human life such as suffering, death, disability, parenting, well-being, and flourishing. This tendency is problematic because it limits the kinds of solutions that can be offered in response to legitimate concerns of relevance to human beings; that is, it promotes technical solutions rather than also social or political ones. For instance, if our concern is confined to the narrow issue of how to use genetic technologies to increase the well-being of our offspring, the answers found will be quite different from those that would be inspired by a more general question about the various ways in which we can increase our offspring's well-being. This tendency is equally worrying because it emphasizes individual solutions to problems, such as how best to ensure the well-being of our offspring, that arguably require, and are thus best addressed by, collective answers.

Third, by challenging mainstream defenses of reprogenetics, I attempt to contest the reductionist view of ethics as an instrument for risk management that underlies most proponents' analyses. Conceptualized in such a way, the goal of an ethical evaluation of biomedical technologies is to address issues related to the risks these technologies pose to, for instance, human health, privacy, autonomy, even parent–child interactions. Ethics thus becomes a tool to help us handle these risks as best we can. If, for instance, we want to determine how best to ensure that reproductive autonomy will be respected or promoted, we should ensure that people can choose according to their values and that, whenever possible, they have access to the technological developments they desire. If we need to determine what mechanisms to put in place to reduce threats to human health that can result from the development and use of reprogenetics, we can ensure that we perform adequate animal experimentation or that we conduct appropriate clinical trials. Of course, attending to risks and to the ways of reducing and managing them is an important aspect of any ethical assessment of technological innovations. But it is not the only relevant aspect. Just as essential are questions about the goals we seek to achieve, the means we find compelling, the ways in which means and ends relate to and shape each other, the kinds of societies we want to live in, and the mechanisms best used to create such societies.

Finally, with this analysis I also want to call attention to the importance of encouraging an informed public dialogue. One of the great needs of our increasingly complex era is to communicate clearly all of the dimensions of scientific and technological advances. Insofar as we are committed to democracy, decisions about what research to fund or what to do with the results of such research cannot be made only by scientists or public policymakers or bioethicists. The advance of biological sciences and technologies presents many wondrous possibilities and some possible pitfalls. It also gives us increasing power over who we and our children are and will be. Because of this, the number and the nature of questions about the direction of our lives and our societies will multiply. The decision-making process must include an informed and engaged citizenry. The challenges presented here to mainstream defenses of reprogenetics are intended to be a step in that direction.

References

Anderson, Elizabeth. 2004. Uses of value judgments in science: a general argument, with lessons from a case study of feminist research on divorce. *Hypatia* 19 (1):1–24.

Asch, Adrienne. 1999. Prenatal diagnosis and selective abortion: a challenge to practice and policy. *American Journal of Public Health* 89 (11):1649–57.

———. 2003. Disability equality and prenatal testing: contradictory or compatible? *Florida State University Law Review* 30 (2):315–42.

Barnes, Elizabeth. 2014. Valuing disability, causing disability. *Ethics* 125 (1):88–113.

Belkin, Lisa. 2001. The Made-to-Order Savior. *The New York Times Magazine*, July 1.

Boorse, Christopher. 1975. On the distinction between disease and illness. *Philosophy and Public Affairs* 5 (1):49–68.

Bostrom, Nick. 2003. Human genetic enhancements: a transhumanist perspective. *Journal of Value Inquiry* 37 (4):493–506.

Caplan, Arthur. 2003. Revulsion is simply not enough: the impending culture war over advances in genetics. *APA Newsletter on Philosophy and Medicine* 2 (2):206–9.

(CDC) Centers for Disease Control and Prevention, American Society for Reproductive Medicine, and Society for Assisted Reproductive Technology. 2014. *2012 Assisted reproductive technology national summary report*. Atlanta, GA: US Department of Health and Human Services.

Code, Lorraine. 1991. *What can she know?: feminist theory and the construction of knowledge*. Ithaca, NY: Cornell University Press.

de Melo-Martin, Inmaculada. 2010. Defending human enhancement technologies: unveiling normativity. *Journal of Medical Ethics* 36 (8):483–7.

DeFrancesco, L. 2014. 23andMe's designer baby patent. *Nature Biotechnology* 32 (1):8.

DeGrazia, David. 2013. Moral enhancement, freedom, and what we (should) value in moral behaviour. *Journal of Medical Ethics* 40 (6):361–8.

Dickenson, Donna L. 2011. Regulating (or not) reproductive medicine: an alternative to letting the market decide. *Indian Journal of Medical Ethics* 8 (3):175–79.

Donchin, Anne. 2010. Reproductive tourism and the quest for global gender justice. *Bioethics* 24 (7):323–32.

Fausto-Sterling, Anne. 1992. *Myths of gender: biological theories about women and men*. 2nd ed. New York: BasicBooks.

Floridi, L., and J. W. Sanders. 2004. On the morality of artificial agents. *Minds and Machines* 14 (3):349–79.

Garland-Thomson, Rosemarie. 2012. The case for conserving disability. *Journal of Bioethical Inquiry* 9 (3):339–55.

Goering, Sara. 2008. 'You say you're happy, but. . .': contested quality of life judgments in bioethics and disability studies. *Journal of Bioethical Inquiry* 5 (2–3):125–35.

Habermas, Jürgen. 2003. *The future of human nature.* Cambridge, UK: Polity.

Haraway, Donna. 1988. Situated knowledges: the science question in feminism and the privilege of partial perspective. *Feminist Studies* 14 (3):575–99.

———. 1989. *Primate visions: gender, race, and nature in the world of modern science.* New York: Routledge.

Harding, Sandra G. 1986. *The science question in feminism.* Ithaca, NY: Cornell University Press.

———. 1991. *Whose science? whose knowledge?: thinking from women's lives.* Ithaca, NY: Cornell University Press.

———. 2008. Sciences from below: feminisms, postcolonialities, and modernities. In *Next wave: new directions in women's studies.* Durham, NC: Duke University Press.

Harris, John. 1998. *Clones, genes, and immortality: ethics and the genetic revolution.* New York: Oxford University Press.

———. 2005. No sex selection please, we're British. *Journal of Medical Ethics* 31 (5):286–8.

———. 2007. *Enhancing evolution: the ethical case for making better people.* Princeton, NJ: Princeton University Press.

Haslanger, Sally. 2000. Gender and race: (what) are they? (what) do we want them to be? *Noûs* 34 (1):31–55.

Hrdy, Sarah B. 1986. Empathy, polyandry and the myth of the coy female. In *Feminist approaches to science,* edited by R. Bleier. New York: Pergamon.

Huxley, Aldous. [1932] 1998. *Brave new world.* 1st Perennial Classics ed. New York: Perennial Classics.

Idhe, Don. 1993. *Postphenomenology.* Evanston, IL: Northwestern University Press.

Jasanoff, Sheila. 2004. *States of knowledge: the co-production of science and social order.* International Library of Sociology. New York: Routledge.

Jasper, M. J., J. Liebelt, and N. D. Hussey. 2008. Preimplantation genetic diagnosis for BRCA1 exon 13 duplication mutation using linked polymorphic markers resulting in a live birth. *Prenatal Diagnosis* 28 (4):292–8.

Jonas, Hans. 1984. *The imperative of responsibility: in search of an ethics for the technological age*. Chicago: University of Chicago Press.

Jordan-Young, Rebecca M. 2010. *Brain storm: the flaws in the science of sex differences*. Cambridge, MA: Harvard University Press.

Kaebnick, Gregory E. 2008. Reasons of the heart: emotion, rationality, and the "wisdom of repugnance." *The Hastings Center Report* 38 (4):36–45.

Kass, Leon R. 1997. The wisdom of repugnance: why we should ban the cloning of humans. *New Republic* 216 (22):17–26.

Keller, Evelyn Fox. 1985. *Reflections on gender and science*. New Haven, CT: Yale University Press.

Kupka, M. S., A. P. Ferraretti, J. de Mouzon, K. Erb, T. D'Hooghe, J. A. Castilla, C. Calhaz-Jorge, C. De Geyter, V. Goossens, and the European IVF-Monitoring (EIM) Consortium, for the European Society of Human Reproduction and Embryology (ESHRE). 2014. Assisted reproductive technology in Europe, 2010: results generated from European registers by ESHRE. *Human Reproduction* 29 (10):2099–113.

Latour, Bruno. 2005. *Reassembling the social: an introduction to actor-network-theory*. Clarendon Lectures in Management Studies. New York: Oxford University Press.

Lloyd, Elisabeth Anne. 2005. *The case of the female orgasm: bias in the science of evolution*. Cambridge, MA: Harvard University Press.

Longino, Helen E. 1987. Can there be a feminist science? *Hypatia* 2 (3):51–64.

Mahowald, Mary Briody. 2000. *Genes, women, equality*. New York: Oxford University Press.

Midgley, Mary. 2000. Biotechnology and monstrosity: why we should pay attention to the "yuk factor." *The Hastings Center Report* 30 (5):7–15.

Mills, Catherine. 2011. The limits of reproductive autonomy: prenatal testing, harm and disability. In *Futures of reproduction: bioethics and biopolitics*. Vol. 49 of International Library of Ethics, Law, and the New Medicine, New York: Springer, 57–83.

Niccol, Andrew. 1997. *Gattaca*. United States: Columbia Pictures.

Niemelä, J. 2011. What puts the "yuck" in the yuck factor? *Bioethics* 25 (5):267–9.

Parens, Erik, and Adrienne Asch. 1999. The disability rights critique of prenatal genetic testing: reflections and recommendations. *The Hastings Center Report* 29 (5):S1–22.

Persson, I., and J. Savulescu. 2008. The perils of cognitive enhancement and the urgent imperative to enhance the moral character of humanity. *Journal of Applied Philosophy* 25 (3):162–7.

Reznek, Lawrie. 1987. *The nature of disease.* Philosophical Issues in Science. New York: Routledge & Kegan Paul.

Roache, R., and S. Clarke. 2009. Bioconservatism, bioliberalism, and the wisdom of reflecting on repugnance. *Monash Bioethics Review* 28 (1):4.1–21.

Rolin, Kristina. 2004. Why gender is a relevant factor in the social epistemology of scientific inquiry. *Philosophy of Science* 71 (5):880–91.

Salles, Arleen, and Inmaculada de Melo-Martin. 2012. Disgust in bioethics. *Cambridge Quarterly of Healthcare Ethics* 21 (2):267–80.

Savulescu, Julian. 2005. New breeds of humans: the moral obligation to enhance. *Reproductive Biomedicine Online* 10 (suppl 1):36–39.

Schiebinger, Londa L. 1989. *The mind has no sex?: women in the origins of modern science.* Cambridge, MA: Harvard University Press.

———. 2004. *Plants and empire: colonial bioprospecting in the Atlantic world.* Cambridge, MA: Harvard University Press.

Scully, Jackie Leach. 2008. *Disability bioethics: moral bodies, moral difference, feminist constructions.* Lanham, MD: Rowman & Littlefield.

Shakespeare, Tom. 2006. *Disability rights and wrongs.* New York: Routledge.

Spanier, Bonnie. 1995. *Im/partial science: gender ideology in molecular biology.* Bloomington, IN: Indiana University Press.

Spar, Debora L. 2006. *The baby business: how money, science, and politics drive the commerce of conception.* Boston: Harvard Business School Press.

Swierstra, T., and K. Waelbers. 2012. Designing a good life: a matrix for the technological mediation of morality. *Science and Engineering Ethics* 18 (1):157–72.

Tingley, Kim. 2014. The brave new world of three-parent I.V.F. *New York Times*, June 27.

Tremain, Shelley. 2001. On the government of disability. *Social Theory and Practice* 27 (4):617–36.

Twine, France Winndance. 2015. *Outsourcing the womb: race, class and gestational surrogacy in a global market.* 2nd ed. Framing 21st Century Social Issues. New York: Routledge, Taylor & Francis Group.

Verbeek, Peter-Paul. 2005. *What things do: philosophical reflections on technology, agency, and design*. University Park, PA: Pennsylvania State University Press.

Wajcman, Judy. 2004. *TechnoFeminism*. Cambridge, UK: Polity.

Wasserman, David, and Adrienne Asch. 2006. The uncertain rationale for prenatal disability screening. *The virtual mentor: VM* 8 (1):53–6.

———. 2014. Understanding the relationship between disability and well-being. In *Disability and the good human life*, edited by J. E. Bickenbach, F. Felder, and B. Schmitz. Cambridge, UK: Cambridge University Press.

Winner, Langdon. 1980. Do artifacts have politics? *Daedalus* 109 (1):121–36.

Wylie, Alison, and Lynn Hankinson Nelson. 2007. Coming to terms with the values of science: insights from feminist science studies scholarship. In *Value-free science?: ideals and illusions*, edited by H. Kincaid, J. Dupre, and A. Wylie. Oxford, UK: Oxford University Press.

Wynne, Brian. 2001. Creating public alienation: expert cultures of risk and ethics on GMOs. *Science as Culture (London)* 10 (4):445–81.

———. 2006. Public engagement as a means of restoring public trust in science: hitting the notes, but missing the music? *Community Genetics* 9 (3):211–20.

Chapter 2

Reprogenetic Technologies

An Overview

Introduction

Although it has been defined in different ways by various authors (Knowles and Kaebnick 2007; Silver 1997), the term "reprogenetics" generally refers to practices that combine reproductive technologies and genetic tools. Strictly speaking, this would include not just technologies such as in vitro fertilization (IVF) and preimplantation genetic diagnosis (PGD) but also practices such as surrogate arrangements and genetic technologies for prenatal genetic testing (e.g., amniocentesis). However, my focus in this chapter and throughout the book is slightly more limited. I discuss here those technologies that allow the creation, storage, and genetic manipulation of gametes and embryos with the aim of reproduction. Of course, these technologies also can be used, and routinely are used, for research purposes. Nevertheless, my concern here is with the use of these technologies to have children.

Some of these reproductive technologies, such as IVF, have been used for almost four decades, although researchers are constantly updating the procedures and techniques involved.

For IVF, these updates include new fertility drugs and cryo-preservation protocols as well as novel techniques such as intracytoplasmic sperm injection. However, the majority of the genetic and molecular tools used in reprogenetics are relatively recent developments. PGD, for instance, was introduced only in the early 1990s, and some of the molecular technologies that can be used today to manipulate the genetic makeup of cells are still in the initial stages of research. In general, reproge-netic technologies have been characterized by their rapid trans-fer from the laboratory to the clinic to routine care—in many cases with scant evidence of safety and efficacy. Moreover, as is common with technological developments, although the initial use of many reprogenetic techniques was limited (i.e., directed toward particular infertility problems or genetic conditions), their application has broadened steadily. Indeed, these technol-ogies can now be used, and are used, in cases in which neither infertility nor the risk of transmitting some genetic mutation is present.

The purpose of this chapter is to offer a brief description of the main reprogenetic technologies in use today and some of the most significant ones being developed. Because of their relevance in the field, I pay particular attention to IVF and PGD. I also discuss the differences between somatic and germ-line modifications and some possible and likely future uses for reprogenetic technologies. I end the chapter with a description of recent technological advances such as mitochondrial transfer and genetic screening of "virtual babies." My goal is not to offer a detailed account of the development and technical aspects of these technologies but rather to provide an overview of what these technologies are and what they involve, with the aim of understanding the ethical issues discussed in the chapters that follow.

Reprogenetic Technologies

In Vitro Fertilization

On July 25, 1978, the collaborating work of gynecologist Patrick Steptoe and physiologist Robert Edwards led to the birth of the first so-called test-tube baby, Louise Brown, in England. Dr. Edwards' contribution to the development of IVF was recognized in 2010 with the Nobel Prize in Physiology or Medicine (Kirby 2010). Since the birth of Louise Brown, approximately 5.4 million babies have been born worldwide with the help of IVF and associated techniques (referred to collectively hereafter as IVF). Although some evidence indicates that the steady growth in its use is slowing, the number of IVF cycles performed, i.e., the process that begins with the stimulation and monitoring of a woman's ovaries with the intent of having embryos transferred, in many developed countries has grown by 5% to 10% annually over recent years (ESHRE 2014). Currently, in several European countries including Belgium, Denmark, and Norway, more than 4.0% of all babies are born through IVF (ESHRE 2014). In the United States, approximately 1.5% of all infants are conceived with the help of these technologies (Sunderam et al. 2014).

IVF, the quintessential type of reproductive technology, was originally developed not as a solution to human fertility problems but as an important research tool for the animal breeding industry to study fertility, embryo development, and heredity issues. It was not until the early 1960s that research on IVF started to focus on the alleviation of human infertility (Chen and Wallach 1994; Perone 1994). In this application, IVF was focused on infertility problems caused by damage to a woman's fallopian tubes. However, it soon became common treatment for a variety of other fertility problems, including inability to produce eggs, poor sperm quality, endometriosis, and unexplained infertility. In its most basic form (i.e., when the woman undergoing IVF provides her own eggs and her husband or partner supplies the sperm), IVF involves several steps (Elder and Dale 2011). The first one, ovarian stimulation, has as its aim the production of multiple oocytes in a cycle. Women usually produce only one oocyte per menstrual cycle. A woman undergoing IVF injects a number of fertility drugs for about 2 weeks in order to increase the chance of collecting multiple eggs. Follicle-stimulating hormone and luteinizing hormone are used to produce as many eggs as possible during a cycle, gonadotropin-releasing hormone to prevent the woman from ovulating too early, and human chorionic gonadotropin to trigger ovulation. These drugs may be used alone or in combination, depending on the cause of infertility and the type of protocol employed (Polat, Bozdag, and Yarali 2014). To monitor the maturation process, the woman undergoes regular transvaginal ultrasound examinations to evaluate the ovaries and blood tests to check hormone levels.

The second step, oocyte retrieval, allows doctors to obtain the matured oocytes before they are released by the ovaries. With the woman under sedation, doctors retrieve the eggs from her ovaries through a transvaginal technique involving an ultrasound-guided probe. A thin needle, which is connected to a suction device, is inserted through the woman's vagina and into the ovary and follicles containing the eggs. The egg and surrounding fluid is pulled out of the follicle, through the hollow tube, and into a test tube. This process is repeated for each ripe follicle in both ovaries. Usually, between 8 and 15 eggs are retrieved. If fresh eggs are to be used, the male partner is asked to ejaculate into a cup so that sperm can be obtained while the retrieval of eggs is taking place. The semen is then washed and prepared in the laboratory.

In the fertilization stage, the eggs are assessed, and those chosen are combined with appropriately prepared sperm in a petri dish and cultured in the laboratory for 16 to 20 hours, after which they are checked to determine whether fertilization has occurred. Often, rather than allowing fertilization in a petri dish, a single sperm is selected, aspirated into the tip of a pipette, and injected directly into the egg, a technique called intracytoplasmic sperm injection (ICSI). Although ICSI was originally developed to improve fertilization rates in cases of severe male factor infertility, today this procedure is widely used even without that diagnosis (Babayev, Park, and Bukulmez 2014). Once fertilization occurs, the embryos are passed to a laboratory incubator containing special growth medium and allowed to grow, usually for 3 to 5 days. The embryologist monitors the development of the embryos and assesses them for transfer. It is at this stage of embryo culture that PGD (described later) can be used to select for particular embryos.

In the last stage, embryo transfer, embryos (usually more than one) are loaded into a catheter, which is inserted through the woman's cervix and into the uterus. Abdominal ultrasound is used to monitor the insertion of the catheter and ensure that it advances to the appropriate location. Once the target location is reached, the embryos are released from the catheter, which is then withdrawn. Women are usually asked to rest for a short period before leaving the clinic. If not all embryos are transferred, those that remain can be cryopreserved for future use. Usually, women receive progesterone injections for about 2 weeks after transfer to aid embryo implantation. About 2 weeks after the transfer of the embryos, a blood test is done to determine whether pregnancy has occurred.

IVF may also be performed with the use of donor eggs or sperm or with donor embryos. Indeed, use of donor cycles has been increasing steadily, and in 2012 donor eggs or embryos were used in 11% of all assisted reproductive technology (ART) cycles performed in the United States (CDC, American Society for Reproductive Medicine, and Society for Assisted Reproductive Technology 2014). In Europe, almost 17% of cycles in 2010 involved the use of donor eggs (Kupka et al. 2014). When fresh donated eggs are used, the cycles of the egg donor and recipient must be synchronized so that the recipient's uterine lining can receive the embryos. Estrogen and progesterone drugs are used for this purpose. The woman providing the eggs follows the ovarian stimulation and oocyte retrieval stages described earlier. After fertilization and assessment, the embryos are transferred into the uterus of the recipient. Women who provide eggs are usually younger than 35 years old. They undergo a number of tests to ensure that there is no evidence of impaired fertility, communicable infectious diseases, or a variety of genetic mutations. They also receive a psychological evaluation.

Interpretation of success rates for IVF is complex because success is affected by multiple factors. When a woman's own eggs are used, age seems to have a significant effect on the chance of having a live birth (CDC 2014). For instance, in 2012 in the United States, the percentage of cycles using fresh, non-donor eggs that resulted in life births was 29% overall. However, for women younger than 35 years of age, that percentage was 40.5%, and for women age 41 or 42, it was 11.7%. When fresh donor eggs were used, the percentage of live births per transfer for women age 41 or 42 years was more than 55%. Other factors, such as the quality of the eggs and sperm, the particular cause of the infertility, the number of embryos transferred, the procedures used, and the woman's history of previous births and miscarriages, also affect the likelihood of IVF success. The training and experience of the professionals at clinics and laboratories are also relevant factors (CDC 2014).

IVF involves not only significant financial resources—the average cost per cycle in the United States is greater than $12,000—but also various risks to the woman's health (Nastri et al. 2015). Each of the steps described earlier involves some health risks.[1] For instance, the fertility drugs used in IVF cycles can cause a variety of side effects including ovarian hyperstimulation syndrome, a condition in which the ovaries are swollen. Similarly, egg retrieval procedures can result in bleeding, infection, and injury to organs near the ovaries, such as the bladder and the bowel. Moreover, a variety of health risks are associated with the multiple pregnancies that usually result from the transfer of more than one embryo (Kissin et al. 2015). Multiple pregnancies also result in increased risks to children (Qin, Wang, et al. 2015) and higher health care costs (Lemos et al. 2013).

Apart from the risks to children of multiple pregnancies, other studies have called attention to the increased health risks to babies born with IVF. Evidence indicates that even singletons born with these technologies are at increased risk of low birth weight, prematurity, and intrauterine growth retardation (Stojnic et al. 2013). Some studies and meta-analyses have also found an increased risk of congenital malformations for infants conceived through IVF (Hansen et al. 2013; Heisey et al. 2015; Qin, Sheng, et al. 2015; Wen et al. 2012). However, it is difficult to determine whether these risks are linked to IVF and associated technologies themselves, or are the result of parental factors such as age or the underlying fertility problems experienced by most couples who use IVF, or derive from a combination of both (Dupont and Sifer 2012; Heisey et al. 2015). More research is needed to assess the effects of IVF on children's health.

---

1. A more detailed discussion of risks associated with IVF appears in chapter 6.

Cryopreservation

Successful cryopreservation of human sperm was achieved in the early 1950s (Bunge and Sherman 1953), and storage of frozen sperm is today a common practice for artificial insemination and IVF. Indeed, with the emergence of HIV/AIDS in the late 1980s, artificial donor insemination has been performed exclusively with frozen and quarantined sperm so that it can be screened for communicable diseases.

Cryopreservation of embryos has likewise been used for a few decades (Trounson and Mohr 1983), and refinement of cryopreservation methods has offered a variety of advantages in the field of assisted reproduction (Wong, Mastenbroek, and Repping 2014). Cryopreservation allows for a decreased number of fresh embryo transfers and thus contributes to a reduction of the risks of multiple pregnancies. It is also crucial when embryo transfer must be cancelled due to ovarian hyperstimulation risks or other unplanned events occurring during the transfer of fresh embryos. Cryopreservation of embryos also allows later use of surplus embryos obtained in a cycle, and therefore it is important for the cumulative pregnancy success rate after IVF. Currently, studies indicate that pregnancy rates are similar or even slightly higher with frozen embryos than with fresh embryos (CDC 2014). Evidence also suggests that health outcomes for children born through IVF are similar with cryopreserved embryos and with fresh ones (Okun, Sierra, and Society of Obstetricians and Gynaecologists of Canada 2014). More studies are needed to assess whether this trend is confirmed in the long term and to evaluate new cryopreservation techniques.

The 1980s saw the first baby conceived with the use of a previously frozen and thawed egg (Chen 1986), but successful births after oocyte freezing have been rare until very recently.

This had to do with technical difficulties in the cryopreservation of oocytes related to their size, their high water content, and the fragility of the chromosomal arrangement (Coticchio et al. 2004). Advances in cryopreservation techniques have now resulted in significant improvements in oocyte freezing (Clark and Swain 2013). In some laboratories, cryopreserved and fresh oocytes show similar rates of survival, insemination, implantation, clinical pregnancy, and delivery (Cil and Seli 2013; Edgar and Gook 2012), but the absolute number of successful pregnancies with frozen eggs is still small. Oocyte freezing was initially thought to be particularly important to improve fertility care for women at risk of losing ovarian function, such as young cancer patients about to undergo chemotherapy or radiation (Noyes et al. 2011). In addition, it can be used for patients who oppose embryo freezing for religious or ethical reasons and for those whose partners are unable to produce semen specimens at the time of retrieval. Cryopreservation also opens the option of oocyte banks that can be used for donation (Mertes et al. 2012).

More controversially, this new procedure is currently being aggressively advertised—some argue with inadequate information (Avraham et al. 2014)—to healthy young women who are said to desire a deferral of motherhood because they do not have a current partner or because of their professional obligations. Indeed, some employers such as Facebook and Apple have decided to include oocyte cryopreservation in their employee benefit packages (Baylis 2015). Given that oocyte cryopreservation protocols are quite new, large safety and efficacy studies are lacking, and long-term safety and efficacy evidence is non-existent, offering this new technology to young, healthy women under the guise of ensuring their future fertility is certainly ethically problematic.

Preimplantation Genetic Diagnosis

Advances in genetic and genomic science and technology during the last decades have considerably increased both our understanding of the genetic basis of human diseases and researchers' ability to manipulate the human genome. The ability to identify changes in chromosomes, genes, or proteins that correlate with particular diseases such as Down syndrome, cystic fibrosis, thalassemia, or Huntington's disease has led to the development of a variety of genetic tests that are now part of routine medical care.

PGD is one of these genetic tests. It was introduced in 1990 (Handyside et al. 1990) as an alternative to prenatal tests for couples at high risk of transmitting monogenic disorders to their offspring. Because our ability to treat or cure many of the diseases for which genetic tests are available is significantly limited, couples who wanted to have children and were at high risk of passing on certain genetic conditions were faced with the options of risking the birth of a child with serious health problems or using prenatal testing and then terminating the pregnancy if the fetus were found to have the mutation in question. Although PGD requires the use of IVF, it was thought to give prospective parents a more desirable option by reducing the chance of having to terminate a wanted pregnancy.

PGD involves the removal, before transfer into the woman's body, of one or more cells from a developing oocyte or embryo in order to test for chromosomal abnormalities or genetic mutations in the genome (Collins 2013). Usually, embryo biopsy is undertaken when the embryo is at the six- to eight-cell stage. A variety of molecular techniques can be used to evaluate the biopsied cells (Simpson 2010). For example, fluorescent in situ hybridization (FISH), a technique that can detect and localize the presence or absence of specific DNA sequences on chromosomes, is normally used for identification of chromosomal abnormalities and for sex determination in cases of X-linked disorders. Polymerase chain reaction (PCR), a technique that allows the amplification of particular pieces of DNA, is normally employed to determine the existence of single-gene disorders, both recessive and dominant, and triplet repeat diseases such as Huntington's disease and fragile-X syndrome. After the cells have been examined, only embryos that are thought to be unaffected are transferred into the woman's uterus.

Until recently, PGD was used mainly to test for disorders caused by chromosomal abnormalities (e.g., Down syndrome), for X-linked diseases (e.g., Duchenne muscular dystrophy, hemophilia), and for single-gene disorders (e.g., Huntington's disease, cystic fibrosis, β-thalassemia, sickle cell anemia) (Harper and Sengupta 2012; Simpson 2010). However, the applications for PGD are rapidly expanding, and approximately 200 different conditions can now be tested. PGD is also being used to assess for some late-onset, lower-penetrance mutations (e.g., *BRCA* mutations associated with hereditary breast and ovarian cancer), to allow sex selection for the purpose of "family balancing," and for human leukocyte antigen (HLA) matching to ensure the birth of a baby who can become a tissue donor for an existing diseased sibling (Brezina and Kutteh 2015). Comprehensive genetic testing techniques such as microarrays and whole genome sequencing, which can screen many chromosomes or genes simultaneously, are currently being evaluated for introduction in the clinic. Such techniques can provide information on hundreds of mutations and variants related not only to disease risks but also to some non–health-related traits (Hens et al. 2013; Kumar et al. 2015).

PGD involves a variety of risks, including the risks of misdiagnosis and of damage to the biopsied embryos, which can result in developmental lag and increased rates of embryonic death before uterine implantation (Brezina and Kutteh 2015; Dahdouh et al. 2015). Moreover, although PGD was introduced as a way to eliminate the risks associated with prenatal screening, such as miscarriage and emotional difficulties related to the decision to terminate a wanted pregnancy, clinical practice recommends subsequent prenatal diagnostic testing via chorionic villus sampling (CVS) or amniocentesis to confirm the results obtained with PGD (Dahdouh et al. 2015). Therefore, the same risks are still present even when PGD is used.

Initial evidence regarding children's health indicates that babies born after PGD show normal neurodevelopment, comparable to that of naturally conceived children (Banerjee et al. 2008; Liebaers et al. 2010). Nonetheless, data concerning long-term health outcomes is nonexistent because PGD is a relatively new technology. Similarly, although pregnancy and birth outcomes for PGD are very similar to those achieved with the use of ICSI (Moutou et al. 2014), ICSI is also a new technology. Therefore, comparison with ICSI pregnancies does not offer information about long-term health effects.

The total utilization of PGD is unknown. In the United States, IVF data are collected by the Centers for Disease Control and Prevention, but information about PGD is not required. The Society for Assisted Reproduction has collected some data on the use of PGD since 2007 (Ginsburg et al. 2011). According to these data, PGD use for single-gene defects and elective sex selection is increasing. The European Society of Human Reproduction and Embryology's Preimplantation Genetic Diagnosis Consortium, established in 1997, also tracks preimplantation genetic testing done internationally, but many countries do not participate (Moutou et al. 2014). The Consortium's most recent report also shows that the number of PGD procedures is increasing. The most common indications were for monogenic diseases such as β-thalassemia and sickle cell syndromes, cystic fibrosis, spinal muscular atrophy, and Huntington's disease.

Virtual Babies

As already indicated, PGD offers prospective parents the opportunity to screen and select created embryos based on information regarding susceptibility to a variety of genetic and chromosomal disorders. However, recent genomic applications are going further. Several companies, including 23andMe and GenePeeks, have patents for services directed at prediction of disease risk (and presumably other phenotypic traits), not of existing embryos but of hypothetical ones (Couzin-Frankel 2012; DeFrancesco 2014). These services are currently being offered to people who will be using sperm or egg donors to provide them with information about their potential children's health. 23andMe, for instance, has patented a software program to calculate the probabilities that a hypothetical child could have a particular phenotypic trait by combining the genotype of a recipient with those of multiple donors. Recipients could specify a variety of traits they wish for their future children, and the program would offer recommendations as to which donors have a higher probability, when combined with the recipient's genome, of creating a child with the desired characteristics. Although screening for many monogenic disorders in donors is now routine, the 23andMe patent includes the possibility of obtaining information about many more monogenic disorders as well as complex or multifactorial disorders such as heart disease, diabetes, and obesity. It also includes information about non-disease traits such as height, eye color, muscle development, expected life span, and athletic endurance (Wojcicki et al. 2010).

Similarly, GenePeeks utilizes software that is said to be able to produce up to 10,000 simulated embryos per pairing of egg and sperm. These are analyzed to search for single-gene mutations related to hundreds of monogenic diseases. This information is then used to provide an index of disease risk in the hypothetical embryo—and child—that would develop from a given sperm–egg combination. The cost of this service is about $2000. Both GenePeeks and 23andMe intend to expand the screening options to include hundreds of traits, from monogenic diseases to complex conditions such as diabetes, Alzheimer's disease, breast cancer, stroke, arteriosclerosis, autism, and schizophrenia, as well as hundreds of non-disease traits such as height; hair, eye, and skin color; breast and lips size and shape, ability to roll the tongue, social intelligence, and cognitive ability (Silver 2010).[2] Although services are offered now to those using donated gametes, the ultimate goal of these companies is to offer the service to any couple wishing to have a baby.

Somatic and Germline Modifications

The genetic technologies previously discussed are directed to prospective parents, offering them information that would allow them to make decisions about selecting those embryos or gametes that are thought to be free of particular disease-related mutations or that have some gene variants associated with other desirable or undesirable traits. However, recent advances in biotechnologies also make plausible the genetic modification of the human genome (Cai and Yang 2014; Carroll 2014).

Genetic modifications of the mammalian genome date back to the 1980s (Carroll 2014). In fact, the use of genetically modified animals has become an essential feature of current biomedical research. Technological developments used for the genetic modification of other animals can in principle be used to modify the genome of human beings. Until recently, many of the available

---

2. Of course, the fact that a patent exists to test for these traits and conditions does not mean that the technical ability to do so exists. As discussed in chapter 5, the ability to develop reliable genetic tests for complex characteristics is questionable.

technologies were unreliable and inefficient, in part because of the difficulty of ensuring accurate additions or deletions of desired candidate genes. Nonetheless, advances in genomic and stem cell science as well as ART make the possibility of at least some germline modifications in humans feasible today (Cai and Yang 2014; Carroll 2014).

Current targeted genome editing technologies using restriction endonucleases provide the ability to insert, remove, or replace DNA in precise ways. They can be used not only to study gene function, biological mechanisms, and disease pathology but also to treat or cure particular diseases (Cai and Yang 2014; Carroll 2014; Richard 2015). These systems have been shown to be significantly more efficient and more accurate than older technologies, and they have the potential to dramatically increase researchers' power to manipulate genomes. Restriction endonucleases allow scientists not just to introduce new genetic material at random places, as older technologies did, but to create specific double-stranded breaks at desired locations in the DNA and to use the cells' own mechanisms to repair such breaks. A variety of engineered nucleases such as zinc finger nucleases (ZFNs), transcription activator-like effector nucleases (TALENs), the CRISPR/Cas9 system, and engineered meganucleases are now being used for genome engineering purposes. They have been employed to modify genes in a variety of organisms, including viruses, bacteria, nematodes, frogs, plants, insects, and fish, as well as mammals such as mice, rats, pigs, and humans. These technologies still have a variety of problems, such as the possibility of cutting at unwanted genome sites, and research is being conducted to reduce them.

Most of the current research with these new technologies has been directed at attempts to modify the genome of somatic cells in order to treat a variety of human diseases, including HIV/AIDS, hemophilia, sickle-cell anemia, and several forms of cancer

(Carroll 2014; Niu, Zhang, and Chen 2014; Richard 2015). Such somatic modifications are not intended to alter sperm and egg cells, so the resulting genomic changes are presumed to affect only the particular individual whose cells have been modified. However, the same technologies can be used for germline modifications, which not only would last throughout the lifetime of the modified individual but would be transmissible via reproduction to future generations. Germline modifications can be directed both to correct genetic mutations implicated in the development of various human diseases and to improve particular characteristics (i.e., genetic enhancement). CRISPR/Cas9, for instance, has reportedly been used already to create genetically modified macaque monkeys (Niu et al. 2014). In May 2015, a team of researchers from China reported on the use of CRISPR to modify human tripronuclear embryos, that is, embryos that result from an oocyte nucleus and two sperm nuclei (Liang et al. 2015). The procedure resulted in a significant number of off-target mutations. Concerns raised by the use of this technique in human embryos led to calls from the scientific community for a moratorium on this type of research (Baltimore et al. 2015; Lanphier et al. 2015). Nonetheless, in February 2016, the UK Human Fertilisation and Embryology Authority (HFEA) granted permission to edit the genomes of healthy human embryos for research purposes (Callaway 2016).

Recent advances in ART have also for the first time opened the possibility of germline modification[3] in human beings through

3. The UK Department of Health has accepted that mitochondrial replacement techniques do involve germline modifications. (The offspring of women, but not of men, who use these techniques will inherit the mitochondrial DNA, and so will future generations.) It has argued, however, that these techniques do not involve genetic modifications. This is so because the Department takes genetic modifications to include only those that alter nuclear DNA (UK Department of Health 2014). This argument has been criticized by leading genetic scientists (Connor 2014).

mitochondrial replacement (Craven et al. 2010; Tachibana et al. 2013). Mitochondria are the cell organelles that are involved in cellular respiration and energy production. They have their own DNA, known as mtDNA, which consists of 37 genes. The mitochondrial genome is inherited maternally; that is, only the egg's mtDNA is passed on to offspring. Although both sexes can inherit mitochondrial disorders, only women are at risk of transmitting the disease to their children.

Mutations in maternally transmitted mtDNA or in genes of the nuclear DNA can affect the ability of mitochondria to produce the energy needed for cellular functions and thus can result in a variety of health problems. These mitochondrial diseases usually affect tissues with a high metabolic demand, such as brain, heart, muscle, and the central nervous system. Symptoms include loss of muscle coordination; muscle weakness; visual problems; hearing problems; heart, liver, and kidney diseases; respiratory disorders; and neurological problems. Mitochondrial diseases are relatively rare, and symptoms are very heterogeneous, but these diseases can be fatal. Because of the difficulty of delivering treatments to the mitochondria, management involves supportive strategies rather than cure.

Recently, groups in the United States and in the United Kingdom have shown the feasibility of creating unaffected embryos by placing the nuclear DNA from the egg of a woman with mutant mtDNA into a donor egg that has no identified mitochondrial mutations (Craven et al. 2010; Tachibana et al. 2013). Mitochondrial replacement techniques (MRTs) might offer women who are at risk of passing on mitochondrial disorders the possibility of having genetically related offspring unaffected by mitochondrial diseases. Two techniques have been investigated: pronuclear transfer and maternal spindle transfer. In the first case, both the egg of the woman with the mutated mtDNA and the egg of the donor with normal mtDNA are fertilized with the intended father's sperm (Craven et al. 2010). The genetic contributions from the egg and the sperm, or pronuclei, are then removed from each embryo. The pronuclei taken from the intended parents' embryo are transferred to an enucleated donor egg with normal mitochondria. This reconstructed embryo is cultured in the laboratory until the blastocyst stage and is then transferred to the woman by the usual embryo transfer techniques carried out during IVF. Because extraction of the pronuclei from the egg that carries the mutated mtDNA can involve removal of some of this mtDNA, the reconstructed embryo may still contain some amount of mutated mtDNA.

In maternal spindle transfer, the nuclear DNA (i.e., the maternal spindle) of a donor egg that has normal mitochondria is removed and replaced with the nuclear DNA from the egg of a woman with mutated mtDNA (Tachibana et al. 2013). Although this technique can also involve carryover of some mutated mtDNA, the smaller size of the spindle, compared with the pronuclei, suggests that fewer mitochondria will be transferred. The reconstructed egg is then fertilized, cultured, and transferred to the prospective mother's uterus.

The UK Parliament, after consultations by the Nuffield Council on Bioethics, the UK HFEA, and the UK Department of Health, voted in February 2015 to approve regulations that permit the licensed clinical use of pronuclear and maternal spindle transfer techniques (HFEA 2015). The new regulations came into effect in October 2015 (*Human Fertilisation and Embryology* 2015), and with them the United Kingdom became the first country to explicitly approve human germline modifications (Torjesen 2014). The HFEA must still develop a licensing framework to evaluate requests from clinicians who want to use mitochondrial replacement techniques in the clinic. Requests will be assessed on a case-by-case basis (HFEA 2015).

In the United States, the Food and Drug Administration (FDA) has jurisdiction over whether clinical trials can go forward using these techniques. An FDA advisory committee met in February 2014 to discuss the animal and in vitro studies that would be necessary to support the safety and the prospect of benefit of mitochondrial replacement technologies before clinical trials could start, as well as the risks to women and children resulting from the use of these techniques and the design of clinical trials necessary to assess safety and efficacy. The FDA requested that the Institute of Medicine (IOM) produce a consensus report regarding the ethical and social policy issues related to MRTs (IOM 2015). An IOM committee met in January 2015 for the first in a series of meetings that took place over a period of approximately 14 months. In February 2016, the committee released a report concluding that it is ethically permissible to conduct clinical investigations of MRTs subject to certain conditions and principles, among them a requirement that initial use of these techniques be limited to the transfer of male embryos in order to prevent potential adverse and uncertain consequences to future generations (IOM 2016).

Conclusion

Reprogenetic technologies include both established technologies used routinely in clinical practice, such as IVF and PGD, and experimental techniques such as those involving the use of genome editing tools. Similarly, some of the current uses of these technologies are common and relatively uncontroversial, such as the use of IVF in cases of infertility or of PGD in cases of severe monogenic diseases, whereas others are newer or more controversial, such as the use of these technologies to select the sex of offspring or to select against diseases involving low-penetrance mutations or late onset. Still other uses of these technologies present serious technical difficulties (e.g., use of genome editing tools to alter the genome of gametes or embryos in order to eliminate the risks of some diseases), are speculative (e.g., use of some of these technologies to change certain physical traits such as eye color or height), or completely fictional (e.g., the ability to genetically enhance a variety of cognitive capacities and character traits such as self-control or empathy). Common to all is the unprecedented level of control in reproductive matters that they afford.[4] It is not simply that reprogenetic technologies permit those who previously might not have been able to have biologically related children to do so. It is that the degree of sophistication of these technologies, together with our growing knowledge of human biology, allows prospective parents to make decisions about what types of children to bring or not bring into the world—choices that were unattainable just a few decades ago.

Proponents of reprogenetics unreservedly support the development and use of all of these technologies. Indeed, even when the scientific community raises alarm about the possible negative consequences of some of them, such as gene editing technologies (Baltimore et al. 2015; Lanphier et al. 2015), advocates reject arguments for proceeding with caution and contend that it is morally imperative to conduct research in order to ensure that these technologies can be used in the future (Harris 2015, 2016; Savulescu et al. 2015). In the chapters that follow, I challenge this enthusiastic and, as I will show, uncritical support for reprogenetics.

References

Avraham, S., R. Machtinger, T. Cahan, A. Sokolov, C. Racowsky, and D. S. Seidman. 2014. What is the quality of information on

---

4. However, as we shall see in chapter 5, this level of control is significantly more limited than what proponents of reprogenetic technologies presume and desire.

social oocyte cryopreservation provided by websites of Society for Assisted Reproductive Technology member fertility clinics? *Fertility and Sterility* 101 (1):222–6.

Babayev, Samir N., Chan Woo Park, and Orhan Bukulmez. 2014. Intracytoplasmic sperm injection indications: how rigorous? *Seminars in Reproductive Medicine* 32 (4):283–90.

Baltimore, D., P. Berg, M. Botchan, et al. 2015. Biotechnology: a prudent path forward for genomic engineering and germline gene modification. *Science* 348 (6230):36–8.

Banerjee, I., M. Shevlin, M. Taranissi, A. Thornhill, H. Abdalla, O. Ozturk, J. Barnes, and A. Sutcliffe. 2008. Health of children conceived after preimplantation genetic diagnosis: a preliminary outcome study. *Reproductive Biomedicine Online* 16 (3):376–81.

Baylis, Francoise. 2015. Left out in the cold: arguments against non-medical oocyte cryopreservation. *Journal of Obstetrics and Gynaecology Canada* 37 (1):64–7.

Brezina, Paul R., and William H. Kutteh. 2015. Clinical applications of preimplantation genetic testing. *BMJ* (February 19):350g7611.

Bunge, R. G., and J. K. Sherman. 1953. Fertilizing capacity of frozen human spermatozoa. *Nature* 172 (4382):767–8.

Cai, M., and Y. Yang. 2014. Targeted genome editing tools for disease modeling and gene therapy. *Current Gene Therapy* 14 (1):2–9.

Callaway, E. 2016. UK scientists gain licence to edit genes in human embryos. *Nature* 530 (7588):18.

Carroll, Dana. 2014. Genome engineering with targetable nucleases. *Annual Review of Biochemistry* 83:409–39.

(CDC) Centers for Disease Control and Prevention, American Society for Reproductive Medicine, and Society for Assisted Reproductive Technology. 2014. *2012 Assisted reproductive technology national summary report*. Atlanta, GA: US Department of Health and Human Services.

Chen, C. 1986. Pregnancy after human oocyte cryopreservation. *Lancet* 1 (8486):884–6.

Chen, S. H., and E. E. Wallach. 1994. Five decades of progress in management of the infertile couple. *Fertility and Sterility* 62 (4):665–85.

Cil, A. P., and E. Seli. 2013. Current trends and progress in clinical applications of oocyte cryopreservation. *Current Opinion in Obstetrics and Gynecology* 25 (3):247–54.

Clark, N. A., and J. E. Swain. 2013. Oocyte cryopreservation: searching for novel improvement strategies. *Journal of Assisted Reproduction and Genetics* 30 (7):865–75.

Collins, Stephen C. 2013. Preimplantation genetic diagnosis: technical advances and expanding applications. *Current Opinion in Obstetrics and Gynecology* 25 (3):201–6.

Connor, S. 2014. Scientists accuse government of dishonesty over GM babies in its regulation of new IVF technique. *The Independent*, July 28.

Coticchio, G., M. A. Bonu, A. Borini, and C. Flamigni. 2004. Oocyte cryopreservation: a biological perspective. *European Journal of Obstetrics and Gynecology and Reproductive Biology* 115 (suppl 1):S2–7.

Couzin-Frankel, J. 2012. Genetics: new company pushes the envelope on pre-conception testing. *Science* 338 (6105):315–6.

Craven, Lyndsey, Helen A. Tuppen, Gareth D. Greggains, et al. 2010. Pronuclear transfer in human embryos to prevent transmission of mitochondrial DNA disease. *Nature* 465 (7294):82–5.

Dahdouh, E. M., J. Balayla, F. Audibert, et al. 2015. Technical update: preimplantation genetic diagnosis and screening. *Journal of Obstetrics and Gynaecology Canada* 37 (5):451–63.

DeFrancesco, L. 2014. 23andMe's designer baby patent. *Nature Biotechnology* 32 (1):8.

Dupont, C., and C. Sifer. 2012. A review of outcome data concerning children born following assisted reproductive technologies. *ISRN Obstetrics and Gynecology* 2012:405382.

Edgar, D. H., and D. A. Gook. 2012. A critical appraisal of cryopreservation (slow cooling versus vitrification) of human oocytes and embryos. *Human Reproduction Update* 18 (5):536–54.

Elder, Kay, and Brian Dale. 2011. *In-vitro fertilization*. 3rd ed. New York: Cambridge University Press.

(ESHRE) European Society of Human Reproduction and Embryology. 2014. ART fact sheet. https://www.eshre.eu/Guidelines-and-Legal/ART-fact-sheet.aspx.

Ginsburg, E. S., V. L. Baker, C. Racowsky, E. Wantman, J. Goldfarb, and J. E. Stern. 2011. Use of preimplantation genetic diagnosis and preimplantation genetic screening in the United States: a Society for Assisted Reproductive Technology Writing Group paper. *Fertility and Sterility* 96 (4):865–8.

Handyside, A. H., E. H. Kontogianni, K. Hardy, and R. M. Winston. 1990. Pregnancies from biopsied human preimplantation embryos sexed by Y-specific DNA amplification. *Nature* 344 (6268):768–70.

Hansen, Michele, Jennifer J. Kurinczuk, Elizabeth Milne, Nicholas de Klerk, and Carol Bower. 2013. Assisted reproductive technology and birth defects: a systematic review and meta-analysis. *Human Reproduction Update* 19 (4):330–53.

Harper, J. C., and S. B. Sengupta. 2012. Preimplantation genetic diagnosis: state of the art 2011. *Human Genetics* 131 (2):175–86.

Harris, John. 2015a. Germline manipulation and our future worlds. *American Journal of Bioethics* 15 (12):30–4.

———. 2016. Germline modification and the burden of human existence. *Cambridge Quarterly of Healthcare Ethics* 25 (1):6–18.

Heisey, Angela S., Erin M. Bell, Michele L. Herdt-Losavio, and Charlotte Druschel. 2015. Surveillance of congenital malformations in infants conceived through assisted reproductive technology or other fertility treatments. *Birth Defects Research Part A: Clinical and Molecular Teratology* 103 (2):119–26.

Hens, Kristien, Wybo Dondorp, Alan H. Handyside, Joyce Harper, Ainsley J. Newson, Guido Pennings, Christoph Rehmann-Sutter, and Guido de Wert. 2013. Dynamics and ethics of comprehensive preimplantation genetic testing: a review of the challenges. *Human Reproduction Update* 19 (4):366–75.

(HFEA) Human Fertilisation and Embryology Authority. 2015. *Statement on mitochondrial donation.* http://www.hfea.gov.uk/9606.html.

Human fertilisation and embryology (mitochondrial donation) regulations 2015. 2015. UK Statutory Instrument No. 572. http://www.legislation.gov.uk/uksi/2015/572/contents/made.

(IOM) Institute of Medicine. 2015. Ethical and social policy considerations of novel techniques for prevention of maternal transmission of mitochondrial DNA diseases. http://iom.nationalacademies.org/activities/research/mitoethics.aspx.

———.2016. *Mitochondrial replacement techniques: ethical, social, and policy considerations.* Washington, DC: National Academy Press.

Kirby, Tony. 2010. Robert Edwards: Nobel Prize for father of in-vitro fertilisation. *Lancet* 376 (9749):1293.

Kissin, D. M., A. D. Kulkarni, A. Mneimneh, L. Warner, S. L. Boulet, S. Crawford, D. J. Jamieson, and National ART Surveillance System (NASS) Group. 2015. Embryo transfer practices and multiple births resulting from assisted reproductive technology: an opportunity for prevention. *Fertility and Sterility* 103 (4):954–91.

Knowles, Lori P., and Gregory E. Kaebnick. 2007. *Reprogenetics: law, policy, and ethical issues*. Baltimore, MD: Johns Hopkins University Press.

Kumar, Akash, Allison Ryan, Jacob O. Kitzman, et al. 2015. Whole genome prediction for preimplantation genetic diagnosis. *Genome Medicine* 7 (1):35.

Kupka, M. S., A. P. Ferraretti, J. de Mouzon, K. Erb, T. D'Hooghe, J. A. Castilla, C. Calhaz-Jorge, C. De Geyter, V. Goossens, and the European IVF Monitoring (EIM) Consortium, for the European Society of Human Reproduction and Embryology (ESHRE). 2014. Assisted reproductive technology in Europe, 2010: results generated from European registers by ESHRE. *Human Reproduction* 29 (10):2099–113.

Lanphier, E., F. Urnov, S. E. Haecker, M. Werner, and J. Smolenski. 2015. Don't edit the human germ line. *Nature* 519 (7544):410–1.

Lemos, E. V., D. M. Zhang, B. J. Van Voorhis, and X. H. Hu. 2013. Healthcare expenses associated with multiple vs singleton pregnancies in the United States. *American Journal of Obstetrics and Gynecology* 209 (6):586.e1–11.

Liang, P., Y. Xu, X. Zhang, et al. 2015. CRISPR/Cas9-mediated gene editing in human tripronuclear zygotes. *Protein & Cell* 6 (5):363–72.

Liebaers, I., S. Desmyttere, W. Verpoest, M. De Rycke, C. Staessen, K. Sermon, P. Devroey, P. Haentjens, and M. Bonduelle. 2010. Report on a consecutive series of 581 children born after blastomere biopsy for preimplantation genetic diagnosis. *Human Reproduction* 25 (1):275–82.

Mertes, H., G. Pennings, W. Dondorp, and G. de Wert. 2012. Implications of oocyte cryostorage for the practice of oocyte donation. *Human Reproduction* 27 (10):2886–93.

Moutou, C., V. Goossens, E. Coonen, M. De Rycke, G. Kokkali, P. Renwick, S. B. SenGupta, K. Vesela, and J. Traeger-Synodinos. 2014. ESHRE PGD Consortium data collection XII: cycles from

January to December 2009 with pregnancy follow-up to October 2010. *Human Reproduction* 29 (5):880–903.

Nastri, C. O., D. M. Teixeira, R. M. Moroni, V. M. S. Leitao, and W. P. Martins. 2015. Ovarian hyperstimulation syndrome: pathophysiology, staging, prediction and prevention. *Ultrasound in Obstetrics and Gynecology* 45 (4):377–93.

Niu, Jingwen, Bin Zhang, and Hu Chen. 2014. Applications of TALENs and CRISPR/Cas9 in human cells and their potentials for gene therapy. *Molecular Biotechnology* 56 (8):681–8.

Niu, Yuyu, Bin Shen, Yiqiang Cui, et al. 2014. Generation of gene-modified cynomolgus monkey via Cas9/RNA-mediated gene targeting in one-cell embryos. *Cell* 156 (4):836–43.

Noyes, N., J. M. Knopman, K. Melzer, M. E. Fino, B. Friedman, and L. M. Westphal. 2011. Oocyte cryopreservation as a fertility preservation measure for cancer patients. *Reproductive Biomedicine Online* 23 (3):323–33.

Okun, N., S. Sierra, and Society of Obstetricians and Gynaecologists of Canada. 2014. Pregnancy outcomes after assisted human reproduction. *Journal of Obstetrics and Gynaecology Canada* 36 (1):64–83.

Perone, N. 1994. In vitro fertilization and embryo transfer: a historical perspective. *Journal of Reproductive Medicine* 39 (9):695–700.

Polat, Mehtap, Gurkan Bozdag, and Hakan Yarali. 2014. Best protocol for controlled ovarian hyperstimulation in assisted reproductive technologies: fact or opinion? *Seminars in Reproductive Medicine* 32 (4):262–71.

Qin, J., X. Sheng, H. Wang, D. Liang, H. Tan, and J. Xia. 2015. Assisted reproductive technology and risk of congenital malformations: a meta-analysis based on cohort studies. *Archives of Gynecology and Obstetrics* 292 (4):777–98.

Qin, J., H. Wang, X. Sheng, D. Liang, H. Tan, and J. Xia. 2015. Pregnancy-related complications and adverse pregnancy outcomes in multiple pregnancies resulting from assisted reproductive technology: a meta-analysis of cohort studies. *Fertility and Sterility* 103 (6):1492–508.e1–7.

Richard, G. F. 2015. Shortening trinucleotide repeats using highly specific endonucleases: a possible approach to gene therapy? *Trends in Genetics* 31 (4):177–86.

Savulescu, Julian, Jonathan Pugh, Thomas Douglas, and Christopher Gyngell. 2015. The moral imperative to continue gene editing research on human embryos. *Protein & Cell* 6 (7):476–79.

Silver, L. M. 1997. *Remaking Eden: cloning and beyond in a brave new world.* 1st ed. New York: Avon Books.

———. 2010. Method and system for selecting a donor or reproductive partner for a potential parent. US Patent 8,805,620, issued August 12, 2014. https://www.google.com/patents/US8805620.

Simpson, J. L. 2010. Preimplantation genetic diagnosis at 20 years. *Prenatal Diagnosis* 30 (7):682–95.

Stojnic, J., N. Radunovic, K. Jeremic, B. K. Kotlica, M. Mitrovic, and I. Tulic. 2013. Perinatal outcome of singleton pregnancies following in vitro fertilization. *Clinical and Experimental Obstetrics and Gynecology* 40 (2):277–83.

Sunderam, Saswati, Dmitry M. Kissin, Sara B. Crawford, Suzanne G. Folger, Denise J. Jamieson, and Wanda D. Barfield. 2014. Assisted reproductive technology surveillance—United States, 2011. *MMWR Morbidity and Mortality Weekly Report* 63 (10):1–28.

Tachibana, Masahito, Paula Amato, Michelle Sparman, 2013. Towards germline gene therapy of inherited mitochondrial diseases. *Nature* 493 (7434):627–31.

Torjesen, Ingrid. 2014. Government gives the go ahead for mitochondrial donation during IVF. *BMJ* (July 24):349g4801.

Trounson, A., and L. Mohr. 1983. Human pregnancy following cryopreservation, thawing and transfer of an 8-cell embryo. *Nature* 305 (5936):707–9.

UK Department of Health, Health Science and Bioethics Division. 2014. Mitochondrial donation: government response to the consultation on draft regulations to permit the use of new treatment techniques to prevent the transmission of a serious mitochondrial disease from mother to child. Published online on July 22, 2014. https://www.gov.uk/government/uploads/system/uploads/attachment_data/file/332881/Consultation_response.pdf.

Wen, J., J. Jiang, C. Y. Ding, J. C. Dai, Y. Liu, Y. K. Xia, J. Y. Liu, and Z. B. Hu. 2012. Birth defects in children conceived by in vitro fertilization and intracytoplasmic sperm injection: a meta-analysis. *Fertility and Sterility* 97 (6):1331–7.

Wojcicki, A., L. Avey, J. L. Mountain, J. M. Macpherson, and J. Y. Tung. 2010. Gamete donor selection based on genetic calculations. US Patent 8,543,339, issued September 24, 2013.https://www.google.com/patents/US8543339.

Wong, K. M., S. Mastenbroek, and S. Repping. 2014. Cryopreservation of human embryos and its contribution to in vitro fertilization success rates. *Fertility and Sterility* 102 (1):19–26.

Chapter 3

Procreative Liberty

The Moral Permissibility of Reprogenetics

Introduction

In 1979, Deng Xiao Ping, who saw population containment as necessary for the success of his economic reform program, introduced the "one-child policy" in China (Djerassi 1980). The policy was met with widespread criticism, both in and out of the country, as a serious violation of the right to reproductive freedom (Alcorn and Beibei 2011; Nie 2014). The ending of the policy in October 2015 received equally broad praise (Hesketh, Zhou, and Wang 2015). Sterilization programs, which were extensive during the 19th century and are still present today, are also widely derided as illegitimate interference with people's reproductive decisions (Reilly 2015). Reproductive choices are seen by most as central to individuals' identities and as a critical aspect of their life plans. Because of this central role, a requirement for a strong presumption against interference with reproductive choices seems plausible.

Reprogenetic technologies are involved directly in many people's reproductive decisions, and their use has been vigorously and enthusiastically defended by well-known authors such as Agar (2005), Buchanan and colleagues (Buchanan 2011; Buchanan et al. 2000), DeGrazia (2012), Harris (2007), Roberston (1994,

2005), Green (2007), and Savulescu (1999, 2001a). In general, proponents of reprogenetics use a right-based liberal approach as the framework to support and assess these technologies.[1] They claim that reproductive choice and parental autonomy are basic freedoms and that interfering with individuals' autonomous reproductive and parental choices is legitimate only when their actions clearly and seriously harm others (Harris 2005a; Robertson 2003; Savulescu 2001a).

As persuasive as appeals to procreative freedom might be in relation to many aspects of reproduction, I argue here that they do little to settle important questions about the permissibility of using reprogenetic technologies. First, there is lack of agreement on the existence, nature, and scope of reproductive liberty. Even if one accepts that reproductive liberty entails the right *to* procreate, further argument is needed to show that such a right also involves the right to have a *particular* child. For that is what reprogenetic technologies aim to achieve. These technologies are used not simply to aid people in having children—to reproduce—but to select or create embryos with certain characteristics that prospective parents value. More often than not, proponents of reprogenetics simply assume, rather than offer arguments, that the selection and enhancement of embryos falls under the scope of procreative liberty. Here, I assess the view that reproductive freedom entails the liberty to use reprogenetic technologies to select or enhance one's offspring and find it wanting. I further argue that even if one were to agree that selection and enhancement fall within the scope of a right to reproduce, proponents' contention that no relevant harms can be proven to result from the use of reprogenetics is unpersuasive.

---

1. This framework sits sometimes uneasily with the avowed utilitarian preferences of some of these authors, such as Harris and Savulescu (see, for instance, Sparrow 2011a). I will put those conflicts aside in this chapter.

One of the most controversial aspects of reprogenetic technologies is that they could be used to select or modify genetic variations that are unrelated to disease, such as sex, hair or skin color, height, or beauty.[2] In assessing the case for procreative liberty, I focus on these uses. I first evaluate proponents' contention that decisions about selecting or enhancing characteristics that are unrelated to disease fall within the scope of reproductive freedom. In evaluating their claims, I focus primarily on sex selection, for two reasons. First, sex selection has been explicitly and vociferously supported by proponents of reprogenetic technologies as clearly deserving of the strong protections associated with procreative liberty. Second, unlike other traits often mentioned in debates about reprogenetics, such as hair or eye color, memory, intelligence, beauty, or height, reprogenetic technologies can be used, and are being used, to select embryos with a particular sex. In 2008, for instance, preimplantation genetic diagnosis (PGD) for sex selection accounted for more than 20% of the use of this technique in cycles with a single indication (Ginsburg et al. 2011). The arguments I present here are, however, applicable to the selection or manipulation of any characteristic not associated with disease.

Procreative Liberty

Advocates of reprogenetic technologies take reproductive or procreative liberty to be well grounded on moral or constitutional

---

2. I am not suggesting that distinctions between disease and non-disease traits or characteristics are clear cut, nor that the concept of disease itself is uncontested, (see, for instance, Boorse 1975 and Reznek 1987). For present purposes, it seems sufficient to concede that there are at least some traits (e.g., hair or eye color, female or male sex) that are usually considered not to involve disease even if variations in some such traits might be "treated" by the medical profession.

bases (Harris 1998, 2005b; Robertson 1994; Savulescu and Dahl 2000). However, whether such a liberty exists and what it entails are matters of considerable ethical and legal debate (Attanasio 1986; Botterell and McLeod 2015; Conly 2005; O'Neill 1979; Pearson 2007; Quigley 2010; Sparrow 2008). That procreative liberty involves a right *not* to reproduce is relatively uncontroversial. Privacy or bodily integrity is usually thought to ground reproductive freedom understood in this way (Dworkin 1993). In the United States, this right has been explicitly protected on constitutionals grounds in a variety of cases, including *Griswold v. Connecticut* and *Roe v. Wade*.[3] But some have argued that reproductive freedom involves not only the right to refrain from procreation—and thus a right to abortion and contraception—but also the right *to* reproduce[4] (Harris 1998; Robertson 1994).

But whether one takes rights to function as protecting vital interests (Lyons 1994; Raz 1986), as giving one control over others' duties (Hart 1982; Wellman 1985), or a combination of both (Sreenivasan 2005), the existence of a right *to* procreate is significantly more controversial than the existence of a right not to reproduce. Disagreements exist, for instance, about whether there are any legitimate grounds for a right so understood, about what those grounds might be, and about the scope

---

3. *Griswold v. Connecticut*, 381 US 479 (1965), struck down a statute that forbade the use of contraceptives on the ground that it invaded the privacy surrounding the marriage relationship. *Roe v. Wade*, 410 US 113 (1973), established that a right to privacy under the due process clause of the 14th Amendment of the US Constitution extends to a woman's decision to have an abortion.

4. This right can be understood as a negative (liberty) right against coercive interference or as a positive (entitlement) right to be provided with the means for its exercise. Although their arguments are not always consistent or sustainable (see, for instance, Mills 2011, Purdy 1996, and Roberts 1995), the authors discussed here usually take the right to reproduce to be a negative right—understood as a right against interference with access to the means of reproduction—rather than a positive one.

of such a right (Botterell and McLeod 2015; de Melo-Martin 2013; Patterson 1999; Pearson 1999, 2007; Quigley 2010). For example, some have argued that the interests most often cited as grounding procreative liberty fail to do so. A genetic or biological interest in reproduction has been defended as supporting the right to procreate (Robertson 1994). But as a variety of authors have correctly argued, such interest is an implausible basis on which to ground a right to procreate for several reasons, including the fact that it would commit one to reject interference with a man's desire to simply impregnate as many women as possible or with a woman's choice to become pregnant simply to experience pregnancy (O'Neill 1979; Pearson 2007; Quigley 2010; Steinbock 1995).

Others have contended that the relevant interest is that of rearing children or becoming a parent (Overall 2012). Although this interest is more plausible, some have also questioned it as grounds for a right to reproduce (Botterell and McLeod 2015; Levy and Lotz 2005). Clearly, people can become parents without engaging in reproduction. Even if the interest in parenting is understood as that of parenting one's biological children, it is not clear that this can serve as grounds for a right to reproduce. Insofar as rearing biological children affords unique experiences, such as rearing a child who resembles oneself or who has one's genes, it is not obvious that an interest in such experiences is worthy of strong protection. If, on the other hand, the experiences afforded by parenting one's biological children can also be had by parenting children who are not biologically related to oneself, it is again not clear why an interest in those parenting experiences would support a right to reproduce.

Similarly, attempts to ground procreative liberty on other, more basic rights, such as bodily autonomy, have also been challenged (Botterell and McLeod 2015; Conly 2005). As mentioned, bodily autonomy can plausibly support a right to *refrain* from reproducing. Clearly, if bodily autonomy means anything, it surely means a right not to be forced to be pregnant against one's will. Some might argue that bodily autonomy or integrity can also ground a right *to* reproduce insofar as people have a right not to be subjected to forced sterilization, abortion, or contraception. But if the concern is bodily integrity, then what is wrong with these practices is that they involve unwanted touching or other violations, not that they prevent someone from reproducing. If so, then a right to bodily integrity by itself is sufficient to protect against all of these practices. Thus it is not obvious that constraints on having children, on how many children to have, or on what means may be used to have them infringes on people's bodily autonomy because none of these restrictions involves bodily violations of any kind.

Sex Selection and Procreative Liberty

As this brief overview of the difficulties surrounding procreative liberty demonstrates, the existence of a right *to* reproduce is certainly not a settled matter. However, as indicated earlier, reprogenetic technologies aim not simply at helping people to have a child but at assisting them in having children with or without certain traits. Thus, even if one accepts that reproductive liberty entails the right *to* procreate, more is needed to show that such a right also involves the right to have a *particular* child. In what follows, I assess supporters' attempts to make such a case. Because John Robertson has offered the most detailed and sophisticated defense of sex selection—and other traits unrelated to diseases—as constitutive of procreative liberty, I focus here on his account.

Robertson's conception of procreative liberty includes both the freedom *not to* reproduce and the freedom *to* reproduce, both of which, he believes, should enjoy presumptive priority in cases of conflict. Given this presumptive priority, the burden of proof is placed on those who want to restrict reproductive liberty to offer compelling arguments involving harm. The reason for this presumptive priority is the existential importance of reproduction for individuals. For Robertson, reproductive decisions are of great significance to human beings because they are central to people's identity, their dignity, and the meaning of their lives (Robertson 1994). Noticeably, though, Robertson takes procreative liberty to involve only decisions about whether to reproduce or not; its protection does not extend to parenting practices. Moreover, Robertson takes genetic relatedness to be essential to the vital interests implicated in reproduction.

Even with these restrictions, procreative liberty, understood as a right to reproduce, is still quite expansive in Robertson's account. It involves not just the freedom to make decisions about coital reproduction that can result in the birth of biologically related offspring, but also the freedom to use available technologies to procreate. Thus, procreative liberty protects an individual's decisions to use in vitro fertilization (IVF), obtain gametes, preserve gametes or embryos for later use, and avail oneself of women who can serve as gestational surrogates (Robertson 1994). All of these activities are related to people's decisions to have offspring. However, Robertson also has been a staunch supporter of the use of reprogenetic technologies to select and enhance at least some embryos' traits (Robertson 1994, 2001, 2003, 2005, 2008). That is, he takes procreative liberty to protect not just decisions about whether or not to have a child but also decisions about having certain children, including whether to have a child of a particular sex. What arguments does he offer?

Robertson acknowledges that not everything that has to do with reproduction implicates procreative liberty (Robertson 1994, 2003). He proposes a test to determine whether a certain procreative decision is protected by the right to reproduce. He calls for an assessment of how closely the reproductive activity in question is connected to avoiding or engaging in reproduction. That is, whether or not procreative liberty entails a right to select or enhance one's offspring's characteristics depends on determining whether such characteristics are central or material to a reproductive decision and thus whether the opportunity to have a child with the traits in question determines whether reproduction will occur (Robertson 1994, 2001, 2003, 2008). For instance, if parents will not reproduce unless they can use sex selection, then, Robertson argues, the activity is constitutive of procreative liberty and therefore deserves a strong presumption against interference. Mere preference for a certain trait will not do, in Robertson's account. For procreative liberty to implicate sex selection, for example, the predilection for a child of a particular sex cannot be simply a mere preference. It needs to be a necessary condition of a decision to have a child at all (Robertson 1994, 1996, 2001, 2003).

Although this criterion for determining whether sex selection is an aspect of reproductive liberty might appear initially plausible, it presents several problems. First, the criterion is insufficient to make a determination about what activities are or are not entailed by procreative liberty. It indicates that a reproductive activity falls within the scope of reproductive liberty if it is tightly connected to a decision about whether or not to reproduce. However, as mentioned earlier, Robertson admits that not all reproductive decisions about whether to have offspring are implicated in the concept of procreative freedom. For instance, he explicitly indicates that home birthing, adoption, and reproductive cloning by persons who are sexually fertile are actions that are closely connected to reproductive decisions, but he believes, nonetheless, that such activities, although they might be protected by other rights, are not protected by procreative liberty (Robertson 1994, 2003). This is so, he argues, because such activities either arise only after reproduction has occurred (e.g., home birthing), do not involve reproduction at all (e.g., adoption), or attempt to achieve something not clearly grounded in our ordinary understanding of why reproduction matters to people (e.g., cloning by people who are fertile) (Robertson 2003).

The rationale to exclude at least some of these activities from the realm of reproductive liberty is certainly puzzling. After all, women might have a very strong preference to deliver at home, and some might choose to forgo reproduction all together if prevented from doing so. Likewise, fertile individuals might have such a strong preference for cloning that, if not allowed to do so, they would choose to remain child free. Be that as it may, insofar as some activities that are tightly related to reproduction fall outside the scope of reproductive freedom, claiming that an activity such as sex selection falls within that scope because it is closely linked to decisions about whether to reproduce or not simply begs the question. What needs to be argued is that sex selection, as a particular type of reproductive decision, is intimately connected to the core interests that make reproduction valuable and is not simply a choice tied to whether to reproduce or not. Robertson, however, fails to provide such an argument.

Robertson does indicate that there is a core of vital interests that give reproduction its value—interests that are exemplified in coital reproduction (Robertson 1994). Reproductive practices that closely advance these core interests are protected under procreative liberty. Although Robertson does not provide much information about what those core interests actually are, he indicates that having normal, healthy offspring, with the intention of rearing and transmitting one's genes to them, is part of such core interests (Robertson 1994, 2003). I believe that Robertson's understanding of the core value of reproduction is problematic for a variety of reasons, but I will put those concerns aside here.[5] Even if one accepts that such interests are central to reproduction, it is not obvious that reprogenetic practices such as sex selection advance what Robertson takes to be the core interests of reproduction. First, clearly, whatever the understanding of "normal" and "healthy," boys and girls can certainly be both. Second, the sex of a child is irrelevant to genetic transmission, and one can meet such an interest equally well by having either boys or girls.

Robertson's criterion requires that people's reproductive decisions involve more than mere preferences. His account, however, is ambiguous about whether determination of the appropriate strength of procreative preferences should be made as a matter of principle or on an individual basis. That is, certain preferences are considered to be appropriately strong a priori because they are thought to advance the core interests of reproduction. For instance, a decision to select for embryos that lack certain genetic mutations related to diseases would be considered to be grounded on an appropriately strong preference because it advances what Robertson takes to be a core value of reproduction, having a healthy child. However, it is not clear how having a child of a particular sex would advance the core values that Robertson defends.

At times, Robertson's language about couples' preferences, their decisions, or their reasons to select for their child's sex (or some other characteristic) clearly suggests that the

---

5. The concept of "normality" is highly contested. Indeed, many proponents of reprogenetics, such as Harris, Savulescu, and Buchanan, have fervently rejected the normative power of the "normal"—even though their positions are arguably incoherent without some such notion (Sparrow 2011b, 2013). The concept of "health" is similarly contested (Boorse 1975; Reznek 1987). Likewise, as I mentioned at the beginning of this chapter, the idea that transmitting one's genes constitutes a core value of reproduction has rightly been questioned.

determination about whether sex selection falls under procreative liberty should be made on an individual basis rather than as a matter of principle. For instance, he often refers to "a couple's willingness to reproduce," or "a couple's decision to reproduce" and talks about couples who have one or more children of a particular sex and might refuse to reproduce further if they cannot use sex selection to achieve gender variety in their family (e.g., Robertson 2001, 2003, 2005). In this instance, we are faced with an epistemological problem: how ought we to conclude that the preferences of a particular couple seeking sex selection are not mere preferences but necessary conditions for reproduction? Clearly, how much money people are willing to pay for a particular choice, how distressed they are about it, or how strongly they express their desire might be indications of the strength of their preference, but these are scarcely adequate grounds to determine whether using sex selection is sine qua non for a choice to reproduce at all. One possible option to test the strength of people's preference for sex selection would be to wait until the end of the couple's reproductive life and see whether they have chosen to reproduce without it. This would indeed provide a good indication of the strength of their preference, but, obviously, it would also be of little help to the couple for whom sex selection was a necessary condition of reproducing. This is not to argue that there is no way to reliably ascertain the strength of a particular preference for sex selection; it is only to point out that it is not such an easy task.

Moreover, even if a criterion were to be proposed to assess the strength of reproductive preferences, who would have the authority to determine that a particular couple's preferences are suitably strong? Leaving this to the couples themselves would obviously do little to limit the types of reproductive decisions that fall within the scope of reproductive liberty. And granting such authority to clinicians would raise a variety of insurmountable problems, not the least of which would be to offer appropriate justification for so doing.

Furthermore, it would seem to follow that, if the strength of one's preference to select a child's sex is what determines whether such a decision falls within procreative liberty and thus must be protected from interference, then the principle of procreative liberty would be inconsistently applied. Whereas the desire to use sex selection would be respected in some cases—because it somehow had been determined that the couple would not reproduce otherwise—in other cases it could be ignored. This would make the right to procreate a very peculiar right indeed.

Finally, why should the strength of someone's preference be relevant at all when determining whether a particular activity is a necessary component of a basic right? Determinations about whether some activity is constitutive of a particular right should be grounded on whether the activity in question is essential to advance the values or interests that the right is intended to protect. Take, for instance, the question of whether money spent to influence political elections falls within the scope of protected free speech. Arguably, such a determination should be accomplished by providing reasons for whether the activity of using money to buy political speech is or is not necessary to promote the values and interests that are protected by a right to free speech. The strength of someone's preference for using money to influence elections—even if that preference is so strong that interfering with it would actually cause the individual to choose not to exercise her free speech right at all—would appear to be irrelevant to the matter under consideration.

If the arguments presented here are correct, then Robertson's criterion to determine whether reprogenetic activities such as sex selection fall within the scope of reproductive liberty fails. How tightly an activity is associated with a decision to reproduce or how strongly it is preferred seems to be either insufficient or irrelevant as grounds for assessing the limits of procreative liberty. What is needed is an account of the value of reproduction for human beings and of the interests that procreative liberty is intended to protect. Insofar as Robertson provides any such account, nothing in it justifies his claims that selection of sex or similar non-disease characteristics is a part of procreative liberty.

Perhaps the issue is not that procreative liberty protects certain vital interests associated with the value of reproduction. It may be that reproductive liberty follows simply from people's interests in being free to make their own choices according to their own values. On this account, reproductive liberty need not be thought of as a fundamental right or as protecting fundamental values related to reproduction. Insofar as reproductive decisions are considered particularly important to people's lives—which seems uncontroversial—then, the argument goes, restrictions on such decisions ought to have strong justification. Something like this seems to be what Harris (2005a) and Savulescu (1999, 2002) have in mind when defending the use of reprogenetic technologies.[6] Harris, whose discussion on this issue offers some detail, calls this "the democratic presumption." According to this presumption, he claims, citizens should be free to choose according to their own values, independently of whether the majority accept such choices and values. For him, only serious and present danger to other citizens or to society justifies interference with citizens' choices. Similarly, Savulescu defends the importance of giving couples the freedom to choose what children they wish to have according to their own values,

---

6. That said, both Harris and Savulescu also often refer to "the right to reproduce." Indeed, Harris (2007, 75–6), explicitly talks about reproductive liberty as a basic human right. However, these authors do not give any account of the grounds for such a right.

even if such choices are disagreeable to others. He thus advocates for allowing people to conduct "experiments in reproduction" (Savulescu 2002, 772). Search as we might in Harris and Savulescu's publications, however, no justification can be found for this concept of overall freedom. They simply seem to take it for granted. But the value of overall freedom is contested. Indeed, one of the authors that Harris cites when defending the democratic presumption, Ronald Dworkin, has explicitly rejected the claim that freedom is valuable as such (Dworkin 1993).

Other than indicating that they should not harm others, Harris and Savulescu say little about what choices should be covered by this democratic presumption. One might find the claim that private choices are good candidates for this presumption convincing, but why should public choices be so protected? Moreover, what counts or should count as a private or public choice is contested (Boyd 1997; Landes 1998). But it is clear that reproductive decisions in general, and those involving the use of reprogenetic technologies in particular, are not at all private decisions. After all, decisions about reproducing are decisions about bringing other people into the world and creating families (Okin 1989). Furthermore, the development of reprogenetic technologies involves funding, training of specialists, and the participation of clinicians and other health professionals. Justification for why decisions that inevitably involve social choices should be thought as deserving of a presumption of liberty are conspicuously absent in the writings of Harris or Savulescu.

Harris (2005a) also indicates that mere preferences do not deserve the same level of protection as choices that involve central issues of value and contends that reproductive choices are more than idle preferences. However, he offers no argument to defend this claim. Even if one were to agree that at least some reproductive decisions (e.g., to have or not have children) are more than mere preferences, it is not at all clear why the desire to have a boy rather than a girl, a child with blue eyes rather than one with brown eyes, or a child with more memory rather than less should not count as a mere preference.

Of course, none of this shows that a right to reproduce is unjustifiable or that reproductive decisions ought not to be understood as deserving of presumption against unwarranted interference. What it does show is that proponents of reprogenetic technologies have failed to offer compelling arguments—or indeed, any arguments at all in some instances—that a right to reproduce entails a right to procreate a *particular* child. Therefore, it is not clear that decisions involving the use of reprogenetic technologies to select or create embryos with traits not associated with diseases should warrant the strong presumption against interference that proponents demand.

The Harm Principle

As mentioned earlier, the rights framework that advocates of reprogenetic technologies use is two-pronged. First, they assert that decisions about selecting or enhancing traits, be they morally significant or morally neutral traits, are constitutive of procreative liberty and thus deserve strong protection against interference. Second, they acknowledge that even when such decisions do fall under the scope of reproductive freedom, such freedom is not absolute. They thus argue that limits to the use of these technologies can be imposed, but only to prevent serious harm to others.

Although, as I have argued, no compelling reasons have been offered to believe that decisions involving reprogenetic technologies are entailed by procreative liberty, I will assume in this section that they have. I will focus here on the issue of harms and show that the "very simple" harm principle that proponents so zealously brandish, even if quite rhetorically powerful, is less useful in the matter under discussion than they acknowledge. Although it is beyond the scope of this work to offer a critical evaluation of the harm principle itself (Feinberg 1984, Hart 1963, Rees 1960, Ten 1980), I will point out some disagreements and ambiguities about its interpretation. My main goal in this section, however, is to call into question the apparent force of this principle when it is used by advocates of reprogenetic technologies. I will show that the harm principle does no real work in advancing proponents' conclusions about the permissibility of these technologies. Instead, they use the enticing appeal of the principle to advance their values and views while avoiding a substantive defense of such values and views. I end by critically evaluating the normative assumptions underlying the use of the harm principle and argue that they are problematic. I will continue to use the issue of sex selection to make my case.

Advocates of reprogenetics rely, either implicitly or explicitly, on the thinking of John Stuart Mill when defending their claims that the prevention of harm to others is the only legitimate grounds for interference with reproductive liberty (Harris 2005c, 2007; Robertson 1994, 2001, 2003, 2005; Savulescu 2002). In *On Liberty*, Mill does indeed defend what has become known as the harm principle, according to which "[t]he only purpose for which power can be rightly exercised over any member of a civilized community, against his will, is to prevent harm to others." (Mill [1859]1978, 9). Reading the work of proponents of reprogenetic technologies, one might be forgiven for thinking that the harm principle is uncontested, unambiguous, or, indeed, "very simple." There are, however, disputes about a variety of aspects related to this principle. For instance, neither Mill nor most other defenders have interpreted the principle in the absolutist way that its strong language might lead one to expect. In fact, it is not clear that Mill understood harm to be either a necessary or a sufficient condition for interfering with someone's actions (Brink 2007; Jacobson 2000). For instance, Mill suggested that sometimes, even if an action results in relevant harm, other considerations need to be entertained in order to determine whether interference with such action is appropriate (Mill [1859]1978, 73). More importantly, he did not seem to object to restrictions on liberty in cases in which individual actions are unlikely to constitute a real and present harm to others, including those that involve the provision of public goods such as education or defense (Mill [1859] 1978, 10, 73, 104–6).

There are also disputes about how to interpret the principle (Brown 1972; Feinberg 1984; Lyons 1979). For instance, whether we construe the principle to restrict all actions that threaten to cause harm or only those that actually do cause harm would have very different implications for liberty. Similarly, more or less constraints on freedom could be justified depending on whether the principle were understood as restricting only conduct that is harmful, or risks harms, to someone or also conduct that fails to prevent harm, or the risk of harm, to others. Clearly, the answers to these questions can produce very different applications of the harm principle. If one understands the principle as justifying interference with a person's actions only for the purpose of preventing that particular person from causing, or risking, harm to others, the restrictions allowed would be significantly more limited than if one takes the principle to justify interference in order to prevent harm, or the risk of harm, to others regardless of who caused the harm. For example, in the case of duty to rescue laws (i.e., laws that punish individuals for failing to aid others in dire need when they could have provided such help at little cost to themselves), these different applications of the harm principle would consider these laws to be either unjustified or justified, respectively.

In any case, one need only read *On Liberty* to see that the society that emerges from Mill's famous work is a highly regulated one. Indeed, it is ironic that Mill actually thought that state regulation of reproductive activity was perfectly justified under the harm principle. In his own, spirited words:

> The fact itself, of causing the existence of a human being, is one of the most responsible actions in the range of human life. To undertake this responsibility—to bestow a life which may be either a curse or a blessing—unless the being on whom it is to be bestowed will have at least the ordinary chances of a desirable existence, is a crime against that being. And in a country either over-peopled or threatened with being so, to produce children, beyond a very small number, with the effect of reducing the reward of labor by their competition is a serious offence against all who live by the remuneration of their labor. The laws which, in many countries on the Continent, forbid marriage unless the parties can show that they have the means of supporting a family do not exceed the legitimate powers of the State; and whether such laws be expedient or not (a question mainly dependent on local circumstances and feelings), they are not objectionable as violations of liberty. Such laws are interferences of the State to prohibit a mischievous act—an act injurious to others, which ought to be a subject of reprobation and social stigma, even when it is not deemed expedient to superadd legal punishment (Mill [1859] 1978, 106–7).

The irony is illuminating. It illustrates the difficulties of brandishing the harm principle as a "simple" way of determining what human activities might or might not be justifiably regulated. In fact, as appealing as the harm principle might be, it is unable by itself to answer a variety of necessary questions. For instance, it cannot tell us why harm matters morally or legally or when it matters: Does it matter only in the case of unconsented harms or also consented ones? More importantly—and this is something that is completely ignored by proponents of reprogenetic technologies—the principle is completely silent about what constitutes harm. This is obviously not a small consideration. If, as some have indicated (Epstein 1995; Harcourt 1999), one can reasonably argue that most, if not all, human activities could be deemed to cause harm to others, or risk doing so, then restrictions on liberty could be quite extensive. This would not only reduce the appeal that the principle has in liberal societies; it would lead to very different conclusions than the ones advanced by reprogenetics supporters. Similarly, in addition to questions about what counts as harm, the principle is also silent regarding who or what might be subject to harm.

It seems, then, that appeals by advocates of reprogenetic technologies to the harm principle are insufficient by themselves. We can very well embrace the principle and nonetheless arrive at very different conclusions than they do. This is so because what does the work in arriving at such conclusions is not the harm principle but other substantive normative assumptions. Without them, the harm principle cannot justify the inclusion of some nontrivial harms and the exclusion of others; it cannot tell us that some harm considerations are warranted but others are speculative. Moreover, the principle is also unhelpful when one is trying to determine what the possible outcomes of certain actions might be, how to evaluate the evidence for harms, and how to balance competing claims of harm. Only when all of these considerations have been determined does the harm principle play a role.

Of course, this is not to say that reasonable responses cannot be offered to all of these issues. But the harm principle cannot provide those answers. Some ethical theory or some vision of the good life must ground claims about what counts or does not count as relevant harm, how to evaluate evidence of harms, and how to weigh them (Harcourt 1999; Smith 2004). And this is exactly what is lacking in mainstream defenses of reprogenetic technologies in general and the use of these technologies for sex selection in particular. Advocates merely invoke the harm principle, as if that were sufficient to make their case. In their defense of sex selection, for instance, proponents acknowledge that certain consequences of such practice could count as harms. Harris (2007, 147), Robertson (2001, 4), and Savulescu (1999, 374) all explicitly accept that, were distortions of the natural sex ratio to result from the use of sex selection, such distortion would count as a relevant harm to consider. Negative health or psychological consequences to the children born through these technologies would also count as potential harms that could justify restrictions. Similarly, Harris (2007, 147) and Robertson (2001, 4) seem to grant that the promotion or reinforcement of sexist practices would be a relevant harm in need of consideration. Savulescu (1999, 374) also appears to acknowledge the promotion of sexism as a potential harm, although in at least some of his writings he has argued that increases in social inequalities, including sexism, are not sufficient to justify restrictions on sex selection and other reprogenetic practices (Savulescu 2001a, 2001b). Other outcomes, however, such as concerns expressed by critics that sex selection involves inappropriately treating children as means to their parents' ends, that such practices might threaten valuable notions of parenthood, or that they might promote commodifying practices, are dismissed by proponents of reprogenetics as inadequate (Harris 2007, 156) or fanciful (Savulescu 1999, 373).

Not only do proponents of reprogenetic technologies claim some harms to be relevant and others irrelevant; they also make determinations about the likely occurrence of such potential harms. For instance, they maintain that insofar as some possible outcomes, such as sex-ratio imbalances, can be thought of as harmful, the harms might not be that bad. After all, they claim, these imbalances could have significant benefits, such as increased influence of the rarer sex and reduction of population growth (Savulescu 1999, 374). Others argue that sex-ratio imbalances—and thus the possible harms resulting from them—are unlikely to occur given the cost and physical burden of using PGD (Robertson 2001, 4). Still others contend that to assume that these harms are inevitable or their effect seriously damaging verges on hysteria (Harris 2007, 147).

But the harm principle cannot be used to make any of these determinations. Other normative assumptions need to be put to work in order to decide that some outcomes of sex selection count as relevant harms while others do not, how serious the harms are, and whether they are likely to occur. By invoking the "very simple" harm principle as the criterion to determine when interference is legitimate, advocates of sex selection ultimately attempt to advance their values and views without troubling to provide a genuine defense of them.

It should be clear, then, that despite proponents' insistence, contesting their conclusions in no way commits one to rejecting the harm principle. One can simply dispute the normative assumptions that underlie their application of the principle. I now turn to such a task by assessing proponents' claims about sexism.[7]

Sex Selection and the Harm Principle

We have seen that proponents of sex selection acknowledge the legitimacy of concerns that allowing people to choose the sex

---

7. Of course, questions about sexism might be irrelevant to the evaluation of other traits. Assessment of the potential harms of selecting or enhancing for other non-disease-related traits would involve other normative assumptions.

of their offspring might increase or strengthen sexist practices. Were this outcome to result from sex selection, constraints on the practice would be thought legitimate at least in principle. However, supporters believe that existing evidence fails to show that the use of sex selection would sanction, increase the risk of, or actually cause the promotion of sexism, at least not in Western societies (e.g., Harris 2007; Robertson 2003; Savulescu and Dahl 2000). What grounds this conclusion? First, it is based on a particular understanding of what constitutes sexism and its harms. Second, it depends on how the evidence is assessed.

Supporters of sex selection seem to conceptualize sexism, either implicitly or explicitly, as the discrimination that results from beliefs or attitudes that one sex is more valuable than, or superior to, the other. For instance, Savulescu and Dahl (2000, 1880) claim that it is unjustifiable to accuse people of sexism if they do not have the "absurd assumption that one sex is 'superior' to another." Robertson (2001, 5) similarly considers sexism as "the assumption that one sex is superior to the other" and the resulting discrimination against members of the supposedly inferior sex. Of course, how one conceives of sexism will shape the assessment of the evidence regarding whether such an outcome is a likely result of sex selection.

Other problematic normative assumptions also play a role in proponents' evaluation of the evidence. For instance, according to reprogenetics advocates, available evidence suggests that, at least in Western societies, those who use sex selection do so for family balancing purposes, to ensure that they have both boys and girls as part of their families (Robertson 2003, 462–3; Savulescu and Dahl 2000, 1880), or simply because they have a preference for sons or daughters (Harris 2007, 146). For proponents, the fact that those who choose sex selection are willing to have children of both sexes indicates that they cannot be motivated by the sexist belief that one sex is more valuable than, or superior to, the other. Similarly, according to proponents, non-prejudicial reasons—presumably reasons that do not assume that one sex is superior to the other—can be given and usually are given by those who choose sex selection, and advocates also take this as evidence that the harm of sexism is unlikely to be an outcome of the use of reprogenetic technologies.

But even assuming that the existing evidence about the use of sex selection shows what proponents claim, what evidence can they present that people's declarations of their motivations are reliable? People are generally guarded about the public pronouncement of immoral beliefs—whether or not they have such beliefs. Moreover, proponents' assumptions also ignore the fact that people can have sexist attitudes that are unconsciously held. Indeed, a significant amount of evidence exists on the phenomenon of implicit racist and sexist bias; that is, biases involving unconscious negative evaluations of others or behavioral responses that show unjustifiable preferences for one group over another (Amodio and Mendoza 2010; Raymond 2013; Wittenbrink and Schwarz 2007). If this is the case, then again people's declarations are insufficient to show that they do not have sexist attitudes or beliefs. Furthermore, it is not clear why we should take people's desires to "balance" their families or the fact that people choose girls with the same frequency as boys as compelling evidence of lack of sexist motivations. Obviously, parents with multiple girls could decide they want a boy precisely because they deem boys to be superior (Wilkinson 2008). Similarly, people could choose individuals of a particular sex even when they firmly believe that the chosen sex is inferior. After all, even "inferior" people can be useful for all kinds of things. Thus, even if one were to accept the conceptualization of sexism espoused by proponents of sex selection, their evaluation of the evidence leaves much to be desired.

But why should we accept this conceptualization of sexism as appropriate? Arguably, as feminist work has shown, sexism is a complex phenomenon that involves not just individuals' beliefs and attitudes but institutional and interpersonal aspects, both intentional and unintentional (Bartky 1990; Davis and Greenstein 2009; Fausto-Sterling 1992; Frye 1983; Haslanger 2012; MacKinnon 1989; Okin 1989; Seavilleklein and Sherwin 2007; Young 2011). A more adequate understanding of sexism would attend to the complexity of such a phenomenon and would consider not just beliefs or attitudes about the superiority of one sex over another as relevant, but also beliefs about the existence of rigid gender roles as well as institutional and social practices that systematically work against women's interests. Under this conception, for instance, beliefs about the existence of behaviors, traits, and attitudes that are thought to be normatively appropriate for women and men by virtue of their being, or appearing to be, women or men and that systematically disadvantage women are also constitutive of sexism. It seems clear that prospective parents' interest in raising a boy or a girl are grounded on their beliefs about the different social roles, behaviors, and practices that are considered appropriate for men and women rather than on any biological aspect (Seavilleklein and Sherwin 2007; Wilkinson 2008). Proponents of sex selection find these preferences unproblematic. In fact, they deem that sex selection practices are legitimated precisely by the belief that raising a girl is different from raising a boy and by the interest people presumably have in these diverse experiences (Harris 2007; Robertson 2001; Savulescu and Dahl 2000). The facts that clinics offering sex selection usually refer to this practice as "gender selection" and that advocates of the practice recognize that gender—and not sex—is what is at stake with this technique (Robertson 2001) only underscore the importance of beliefs about gender roles in the use of sex selection techniques.

When one conceptualizes sexism in this more complex way, it is more difficult to argue that sex selection is not the result of sexist beliefs and attitudes or that it is unlikely to contribute to reinforcement of sexist practices. It would be hard, for example, to dismiss the considerable amount of evidence that rigid gender expectations have historically been used to limit the life options of men and particularly of women. It would be equally difficult to discard the evidence showing that the traditional expectations that attach to standard gender roles are related to existing patterns of gender discrimination and sexual oppression (Brandt 2011; Carnes, Morrissey, and Geller 2008; Davis and Greenstein 2009; Economic and Social Council 2010; European Commission 2009; Zhuge et al. 2011). Moreover, still today, social and institutional practices are grounded on gender expectations that are at least in part responsible for limiting the number of women in a variety of career paths, such as the physical sciences and engineering. These expectations ground policies that disadvantage women, such as those regarding family leave and tenure or promotion criteria, and they are the basis for norms about activities as relevant to a person's well-being as child care, household responsibilities, and caring for the old and the sick (Brandt 2011; Carnes, Morrissey, and Geller 2008; Davis and Greenstein 2009; Economic and Social Council 2010; European Commission 2009; Zhuge et al. 2011).

Arguably, the consolidation—through the blessing of modern science and medicine, no less—of rigid gender expectations can only serve to perpetuate this limitation of life choices and to further injustice. Focusing only on the beliefs or attitudes of prospective parents when assessing whether sex selection might reinforce sexism is inadequate. Conceptualizing the problem of sexism and its consequences mainly as the result of individual psychological factors is as best simplistic, at worst completely mistaken. Historical, organizational, and linguistic practices are part of the problem of sexism, and particular institutional arrangements and policies that involve subtle discriminatory practices have much to do with its pervading presence. Thus, even if one accepts that sexist practices cannot exist if no particular individual holds sexist motives or attitudes, the view that sexism and the problems resulting from it are simply the result of individual psychology is highly problematic. Insofar as sexism is the result of structural factors, focusing only on whether prospective parents hold sexist beliefs or attitudes is hardly sufficient.

Concerns about sex selection can extend not only to the negative effects of this practice on women's lives and on society. One can reasonably argue that problematic beliefs about rigid gender roles that underlie sex selection can also result in harms to the individual children born through this technique.[8] This argument calls attention not to the harms that might result from sexist beliefs that I have already discussed (e.g., limitations of opportunities in one's life) but to those that can result from the fact that prospective parents may fail to have the child they are hoping for (i.e., a child who behaves according to expected gender norms). After all, what reprogenetic technologies can offer is the selection of an embryo carrying XX or XY chromosomes. It cannot deliver a child who would behave according to the attitudes, behaviors, and roles often associated with a particular gender. As proponents of sex selection readily concede, however, a child of a particular *gender* is precisely what parents choosing sex selection ultimately want. Whatever the relationships between biological sex and the normative psychological and behavioral characteristics associated with a particular gender, it is clear that biology is

---

8. I am not arguing that these harms, were they shown to exist, are sufficient to warrant interferences with sex selection. My contention here is simply that proponents' arguments fail to show that these considerations are completely irrelevant or that these harms would be nonexistent.

not determinative of gender characteristics (Butler 2004; Caplan and Caplan 2009; Fausto-Sterling 1992, 2000). Indeed, as is well known, even chromosomal sex is only an aspect of biological sex (Öçal 2011), and as the existence of intersexuals, trans-sexuals, and transvestites shows, neither chromosomal sex nor other aspects of biological sex are guarantors of gender (Fausto-Sterling 2000). Moreover, ample evidence shows that chromosomal sex does not guarantee a particular sexual orientation, one of the traits most often associated with gender.

Advocates of sex selection have responded to this concern in two different ways. In some instances, they insist that there are no good reasons to believe that prospective parents who use sex selection would not come to love their children even if they do not fulfill the parents' gender role expectations (Robertson 2001). They contend that parents often have hopes and expectations for their children that go unfulfilled but that nonetheless most parents come to accept and love their children the way they are (Green 2007; Savulescu 1999). This might be so, but it is at least equally plausible to believe that prospective parents who presumably would not have reproduced had it not been for the option to use sex selection, and who have spent the amount of time, energy, money, and health risks that sex selection requires in order to have a child of a particular sex, are not going to be particularly accepting if the child fails to fulfill their preconceived gender expectations. After all, it is not that we do not have any evidence of parents' rejecting children who do not meet gender expectations.

In other cases, proponents of sex selection have deemed that considerations of harms to offspring are irrelevant because of the non-identity problem (Harris 2007; Robertson 2003; Savulescu 1999). According to the non-identity problem (Parfit 1984), because the particular child in question would not have been born had it not been for the possibility of using sex selection, it is at least not obvious that the child has been harmed by the selection of his or her sex. Insofar as the child's life will be worth living, it is not evident that the child can be said to have been harmed given that the alternative would be nonexistence. However, even if one accepts that the non-identity problem calls into question the validity of arguments about harms to offspring in the context of reprogenetics,[9] it is not clear that concerns about the welfare of offspring are irrelevant in this context. The harms to consider here are not those related to creating a boy or a girl but harms that would result from lack of acceptance of the parents if the child does not meet their gender expectations. The comparison here is not with nonexistence but with having parents who love and accept their child.

Notice that the harm principle does no work whatsoever in the preceding discussion. No possible use of the harm principle could tell us that we must conceive of sexism either as simply involving individuals' beliefs or attitudes about the superiority of one sex or as a more complex phenomenon comprising institutional and interpersonal aspects, both intentional and unintentional. And no possible application of the harm principle could tell us how to assess the evidence regarding whether sex selection practices might promote or reinforce sexism in our societies.

It seems, then, that the appeal by advocates of sex selection to the harm principle is less than successful. First, it is not clear that harm to others is either a necessary or a sufficient condition for legitimate interference with people's liberties. Second, one can endorse the harm principle and still question proponents' conclusions regarding sex selection. This is so because the

---

9. It is beyond the scope of this chapter to evaluate the non-identity problem, a problem for which a variety of solutions have been offered. But not everyone accepts that a child who would not have existed but for the option of choosing a particular trait cannot have been harmed (see, for instance, Harman 2004). See also chapter 4 for further discussion related to the non-identity problem.

harm principle tells us nothing about what counts as a harm, how to understand the harm in question, or how to compare, balance, or judge the seriousness of different harms. Third, if one dismisses all these difficulties with the harm principle and acknowledges that other value considerations are at stake when determining whether sex selection practices can result in harmful effects, then it is difficult to see how one can reject the reasonableness of claims that at least some nontrivial harms are likely to result from the use of sex selection. Of course, such a conclusion might not necessarily show that the practice should be regulated because the harms of regulation need also to be taken into account. But on this, too, the harm principle is silent.

Conclusion

I have here called into question the framework of procreative liberty that advocates of reprogenetic technologies often use to defend their position. I have argued that whether there is a right to reproduce and what that right entails are contested issues. Even if one were to accept that the right *to* reproduce ought to have strong protections against interference, proponents offer no compelling reasons for their claim that use of reprogenetic technologies to select or modify genetic variations that are unrelated to disease (e.g., sex) falls within the scope of procreative liberty. They beg the question, problematically ground reproductive rights on the strength of preferences, or implausibly take reproductive choices as primarily private ones. But if decisions involving selection or modification of embryos for non–disease-related traits cannot be properly said to fall within the scope of procreative liberty, then advocates fail to be persuasive when they claim that the only legitimate reason to interfere with the use of this practice is to prevent harm to others. Nonetheless, I have also considered the option that reproductive decisions about selection or enhancement do indeed fall within the scope of procreative liberty and that the only legitimate reason to limit these activities would be harm to others. However, a careful examination of the "very simple" harm principle establishes that the principle is not that simple after all. Indeed, rejecting proponents' conclusions about the permissibility of regulating reprogenetic technologies in no way commits one to rejecting the harm principle. This is so because the principle is mute regarding what counts as a harm, how to conceptualize possible harms, and how to assess the likelihood that certain harmful outcomes would come to pass. Such determinations are grounded on other substantive normative assumptions that proponents simply take for granted, many of which are not only unsupported and implausible but also decidedly problematic.

References

Agar, Nicholas. 2005. *Liberal eugenics: in defence of human enhancement*. Malden, MA: Blackwell Publishing.

Alcorn, T., and B. Beibei. 2011. China's fertility policy persists, despite debate. *Lancet* 378 (9802):1539–40.

Amodio, D. M., and S. A. Mendoza. 2010. Implicit intergroup bias: cognitive, affective, and motivational underpinnings. In *Handbook of Implicit Social Cognition*, edited by B. Gawronski and B. K. Payne. New York: The Guilford Press.

Attanasio, J. B. 1986. The constitutionality of regulating human genetic-engineering: where procreative liberty and equal-opportunity collide. *University of Chicago Law Review* 53 (4):1274–342.

Bartky, Sandra Lee. 1990. *Femininity and domination: studies in the phenomenology of oppression*. Thinking Gender. New York: Routledge.

Boorse, Christopher. 1975. On the distinction between disease and illness. *Philosophy and Public Affairs* 5:49–68.

Botterell, Andrew, and Carolyn McLeod. 2015. Can a right to reproduce justify the status quo on parental licensing? In *Permissible progeny?: the morality of procreation and parenting*, edited by S. Hannan, S. Brennan, and R. Vernon. New York: Oxford University Press.

Boyd, Susan B. 1997. *Challenging the public/private divide: feminism, law, and public policy.* Toronto: University of Toronto Press.

Brandt, M. J. 2011. Sexism and gender inequality across 57 societies. *Psychological Science* 22 (11):1413–18.

Brink, D. 2014. Mill's moral and political philosophy. In *Stanford Encyclopedia of Philosophy*, edited by E. N. Zalta. http://plato.stanford.edu/archives/fall2014/entries/mill-moral-political

Brown, D. G. 1972. Mill on liberty and morality. *Philosophical Review* 81 (2):133–58.

Buchanan, Allen E. 2011. *Beyond humanity?: the ethics of biomedical enhancement.* Uehiro Series in Practical Ethics. New York: Oxford University Press.

Buchanan, Allen E., Dan W. Brock, Norman Daniels, and Daniel Wikler. 2000. *From chance to choice: genetics and justice.* New York: Cambridge University Press.

Butler, Judith. 2004. *Undoing gender.* New York: Routledge.

Caplan, Paula J., and Jeremy B. Caplan. 2009. *Thinking critically about research on sex and gender.* 3rd ed. Boston: Pearson/Allyn and Bacon.

Carnes, M., C. Morrissey, and S. E. Geller. 2008. Women's health and women's leadership in academic medicine: hitting the same glass ceiling? *Journal of Women's Health* 17 (9):1453–62.

Conly, S. 2005. The right to procreation: merits and limits. *American Philosophical Quarterly* 42 (2):105–15.

Davis, S. N., and T. N. Greenstein. 2009. Gender ideology: components, predictors, and consequences. *Annual Review of Sociology* 35:87–105.

de Melo-Martin, Inmaculada. 2013. Sex selection and the procreative liberty framework. *Kennedy Institute of Ethics Journal* 23(1):1–18.

DeGrazia, David. 2012. *Creation ethics: reproduction, genetics, and quality of life.* New York: Oxford University Press.

Djerassi, C. 1980. The politics of contraception: the view from Beijing. *New England Journal of Medicine* 303 (6):334–6.

Dworkin, Ronald. 1993. *Life's dominion: an argument about abortion, euthanasia, and individual freedom.* New York: Knopf.

Economic and Social Council, United Nations. 2010. *Achieving gender equality and women's empowerment and strengthening development cooperation*. New York: United Nations Department of Economic and Social Affairs, Office for ECOSOC Support and Coordination.

Epstein, R.A. 1995. The harm principle–and how it grew. *The University of Toronto Law Journal* 45 (4):369–417.

European Commission. 2009. *She figures 2009: statistics and indicators on gender equality in science*. EU 23856 EN. Brussels: European Commission Directorate-General for Research.

Fausto-Sterling, Anne. 1992. *Myths of gender: biological theories about women and men*. 2nd ed. New York: BasicBooks.

———. 2000. *Sexing the body: gender politics and the construction of sexuality*. 1st ed. New York: Basic Books.

Feinberg, Joel. 1984. *The moral limits of the criminal law*. 4 vols. New York: Oxford University Press.

Frye, Marilyn. 1983. *The politics of reality: essays in feminist theory*. The Crossing Press Feminist Series. Trumansburg, NY: Crossing Press.

Ginsburg, E. S., V. L. Baker, C. Racowsky, E. Wantman, J. Goldfarb, and J. E. Stern. 2011. Use of preimplantation genetic diagnosis and preimplantation genetic screening in the United States: a Society for Assisted Reproductive Technology Writing Group paper. *Fertility and Sterility* 96 (4):865–8.

Green, Ronald Michael. 2007. *Babies by design: the ethics of genetic choice*. New Haven, CT: Yale University Press.

Harcourt, B. E. 1999. The collapse of the harm principle. *Journal of Criminal Law and Criminology* 90 (1):109–94.

Harman, E. 2004. Can we harm and benefit in creating? *Philosophical Perspectives* 18 (1):89–113.

Harris, John. 1998. Rights and reproductive choice. In *The future of human reproduction*, edited by J. Harris and S. Holm. Oxford, UK: Oxford University Press.

———. 2005a. No sex selection please, we're British. *Journal of Medical Ethics* 31 (5):286–8.

———. 2005b. Reproductive liberty, disease and disability. *Reproductive Biomedicine Online* 10 (suppl 1):13–6.

———. 2005c. Sex selection and regulated hatred. *Journal of Medical Ethics* 31 (5):291–4.

———. 2007. *Enhancing evolution: the ethical case for making better people*. Princeton, NJ: Princeton University Press.

Hart, H. L. A. 1963. *Law, liberty, and morality*. Stanford, CA: Stanford University Press.

———. 1982. *Essays on Bentham: studies in jurisprudence and political theory*. New York: Oxford University Press.

Haslanger, Sally Anne. 2012. *Resisting reality: social construction and social critique*. New York: Oxford University Press.

Hesketh, T., X. Zhou, and Y. Wang. 2015. The end of the ne-child policy: lasting implications for China. *JAMA* 314 (24):2619–20.

Jacobson, D. 2000. Mill on liberty, speech, and the free society. *Philosophy and Public Affairs* 29 (3):276–309.

Landes, Joan B. 1998. *Feminism, the public and the private*. Oxford Readings in Feminism. New York: Oxford University Press.

Levy, N., and M. Lotz. 2005. Reproductive cloning and a (kind of) genetic fallacy. *Bioethics* 19 (3):232–50.

Lyons, D. 1979. Liberty and harm to others. *Canadian Journal of Philosophy* 5:1–19.

———. 1994. *Rights, welfare, and Mill's moral theory*. New York: Oxford University Press.

MacKinnon, Catharine A. 1989. *Toward a feminist theory of the state*. Cambridge, MA: Harvard University Press.

Mill, John Stuart. [1859] 1978. *On liberty*, edited by E. Rapaport. Indianapolis, IN: Hackett Publishing Company.

Mills, C. 2011. The limits of reproductive autonomy: prenatal testing, harm and disability. In *Futures of reproduction: bioethics and biopolitics*. 2nd ed., 57–83. Vol 49 of International Library of Ethics, Law, and the New Medicine. New York: Springer.

Nie, J. B. 2014. China's one-child policy, a policy without a future: pitfalls of the "common good" argument and the authoritarian model. *Cambridge Quarterly of Healthcare Ethics* 23 (3):272–87.

Öçal, G. 2011. Current concepts in disorders of sexual development. *Journal of Clinical Research in Pediatric Endocrinology* 3 (3):105–14.

O'Neill, Onora. 1979. Begetting, bearing, and rearing. In *Having children: philosophical and legal reflections on parenthood*, edited by O. O'Neill and W. Ruddick. New York: Oxford University Press.

Okin, Susan Moller. 1989. *Justice, gender, and the family*. New York: Basic Books.

Overall, Christine. 2012. *Why have children?: the ethical debate*. Basic Bioethics. Cambridge, MA: MIT Press.

Parfit, Derek. 1984. *Reasons and persons*. Oxford, UK: Clarendon Press.

Patterson, T. S. 1999. The outer limits of human genetic engineering: a constitutional examination of parents' procreative liberty to genetically enhance their offspring. *Hastings Constitutional Law Quarterly* 26 (4):913–33.

Pearson, Y. E. 2007. Storks, cabbage patches, and the right to procreate. *Journal of Bioethical Inquiry* 4 (2):105–15.

Purdy, Laura M. 1996. *Reproducing persons: issues in feminist bioethics*. Ithaca, NY: Cornell University Press.

Quigley, M. 2010. A right to reproduce? *Bioethics* 24 (8):403–11.

Raymond, Jennifer. 2013. Most of us are biased. *Nature* 495 (7439):33–4.

Raz, Joseph. 1986. *The morality of freedom*. New York: Oxford University Press.

Rees, J.C. 1960. A re-reading of Mill on liberty. *Political Studies* 8 (2):113–129.

Reilly, P. R. 2015. Eugenics and involuntary sterilization: 1907–2015. *Annual Review of Genomics and Human Genetics* 16:351–68.

Reznek, Lawrie. 1987. *The nature of disease*. Philosophical Issues in Science. London; New York: Routledge & Kegan Paul.

Roberts, D. E. 1995. Social justice, procreative liberty, and the limits of liberal theory: Robertson's "Children of Choice." *Law and Social Inquiry* 20 (4):1005–21.

Robertson, John A. 1994. *Children of choice: freedom and the new reproductive technologies*. Princeton, NJ: Princeton University Press.

———. 1996. Genetic selection of offspring characteristics. *Boston University Law Review* 76 (3):421–82.

———. 2001. Preconception gender selection. *American Journal of Bioethics* 1 (1):2–9.

———. 2003. Procreative liberty in the era of genomics. *American Journal of Law and Medicine* 29 (4):439–87.

———. 2005. Ethics and the future of preimplantation genetic diagnosis. *Reproductive Biomedicine Online* 10 (suppl 1):97–101.

———. 2008. Assisting reproduction, choosing genes, and the scope of reproductive freedom. *George Washington Law Review* 76 (6):1490–1513.

Savulescu, Julian. 1999. Sex selection: the case for. *Medical Journal of Australia* 171 (7):373–5.

———. 2001a. In defense of selection for nondisease genes. *American Journal of Bioethics* 1 (1):16–9.

————. 2001b. Procreative beneficence: why we should select the best children. *Bioethics* 15 (5–6):413–26.

————. 2002. Education and debate: deaf lesbians, "designer disability," and the future of medicine. *BMJ* 325 (7367):771–3.

Savulescu, J., and E. Dahl. 2000. Sex selection and preimplantation diagnosis: a response to the Ethics Committee of the American Society of Reproductive Medicine. *Human Reproduction* 15 (9):1879–80.

Seavilleklein, V., and S. Sherwin. 2007. The myth of the gendered chromosome: sex selection and the social interest. *Cambridge Quarterly of Healthcare Ethics* 16 (1):7–19.

Smith, S. D. 2004. The hollowness of the harm principle. *University of San Diego School of Law Public Law and Legal Theory Research Paper Series* 17:1–56.

Sparrow, Robert. 2008. Is it "every man's right to have babies if he wants them"? Male pregnancy and the limits of reproductive liberty. *Kennedy Institute of Ethics Journal* 18 (3):275–99.

————. 2011a. A not-so-new eugenics: Harris and Savulescu on human enhancement. *Hastings Center Report* 41 (1):32–42.

————. 2011b. Harris, harmed states, and sexed bodies. *J Med Ethics* 37 (5):276–9.

————. 2013. Queerin' the PGD clinic: human enhancement and the future of bodily diversity. *Journal of Medical Humanities* 34 (2):177–96.

Sreenivasan, G. 2005. A hybrid theory of claim-rights. *Oxford Journal of Legal Studies* 25:257–74.

Steinbock, B. 1995. A philosopher looks at assisted reproduction. *Journal of Assisted Reproduction and Genetics* 12 (8):543–51.

Ten, C. L. 1980. *Mill on liberty.* Oxford, UK: Clarendon Press.

Wellman, Carl. 1985. *A theory of rights: persons under laws, institutions, and morals.* Totowa, NJ: Rowman & Allanheld.

Wilkinson, S. 2008. Sexism, sex selection and "family balancing." *Medical Law Review* 16 (3):369–89.

Wittenbrink, Bernd, and Norbert Schwarz. 2007. *Implicit measures of attitudes.* New York: Guilford Press.

Young, Iris Marion. 2011. *Responsibility for justice.* Oxford Political Philosophy. New York: Oxford University Press.

Zhuge, Y., J. Kaufman, D. M. Simeone, H. Chen, and O. C. Velazquez. 2011. Is there still a glass ceiling for women in academic surgery? *Annals of Surgery* 253 (4):637–43.

Chapter 4

Conscripted in the Pursuit of Perfection

The Moral Obligation to use Reprogenetic Technologies

Introduction

In chapter 3, we saw that proponents of reprogenetic technologies defend the *moral permissibility* of using these techniques both to select and to enhance embryos with particular traits unrelated to disease. Some of these proponents have gone further and have made the stronger claim that use of these technologies is in fact *morally required*. Savulescu (2001a, 2001b; Savulescu and Kahane 2009), for instance, is well known for his defense of a moral obligation to use reprogenetic technologies in order to select the child who is expected to have the best life prospects. Both Savulescu (2005) and Harris (2007, 2009) have also advocated for a moral duty to use these technologies for enhancement purposes. In this chapter, I tackle the defense of these putative moral obligations. Because the arguments that these authors have given for the existence of these two moral obligations—to select and to enhance—have different grounds, I discuss them separately. I first present the arguments for the putative moral obligation that prospective parents have to select particular embryos and call its existence into question. I then discuss the arguments supporting a moral duty to enhance, and I again find them wanting. The arguments offered in favor of these two moral duties suffer from a host of problems, and it would require more than a chapter to discuss all of them. Many of those problems have been amply discussed elsewhere (Bennett 2009; de Melo-Martin 2004; Elster 2011; Herissone-Kelly 2006; Holm and Bennett 2014; Parker 2007; Sparrow 2011, 2012; Stoller 2008). Therefore, instead of aiming to provide a comprehensive account of all such problems, I focus only on those that I take to be more devastating for these moral duties.

Procreative Beneficence: The Moral Obligation to Select the Best Child

In 2001, Savulescu first offered his defense of what he called the principle of "procreative beneficence" (PB). He presented the principle as follows:

> Couples (or single reproducers) should select the child, of the possible children they could have, who is expected to have the best life, or at least as good a life as the others, based on the relevant, available information (Savulescu 2001b, 415).

His goal in that article was not simply to defend PB but to argue that the principle entails the requirement that prospective parents avail themselves of information both about genetic mutations related to disease states and also about genetic variants unrelated to diseases, such as intelligence, memory, or sex. According to Savulescu, the main reason for including selection of non-disease gene variants as part of prospective parents' moral obligations is that it is not disease that is important but the impact of the genes on well-being (Savulescu 2001b, 423).

Thus, he argued, insofar as non-disease variants such as those related to cognitive capacities or physical appearance affect an individual's well-being, parents have an obligation to acquire such information and select accordingly. He insisted that this is a moral rather than a legal obligation and therefore that persuasion is justified but coercion is not warranted. In that first article defending PB, he also explicitly argued that the moral obligation to select the best child obtains even if fulfilling it maintains or increases social inequality.

PB has received numerous criticisms on multiple grounds, including its theoretical underpinnings and its problematic consequences. Although I believe that many of the criticisms leveled against PB are fatal, Savulescu (2007), sometimes in collaboration with other colleagues (Savulescu and Kahane 2009), has continued to defend it. In the process, PB has been reformulated. In the most recent articulation, Savulescu and Kahane offered the following version:

> If couples (or single reproducers) have decided to have a child, and selection is possible, then they have a significant moral reason to select the child, of the possible children they could have, whose life can be expected, in light of the relevant available information, to go best or at least not worse than any of the others (Savulescu and Kahane 2009, 274).

As should be obvious, the differences in the two formulations of the principle are quite relevant. Although not acknowledged by Savulescu and colleagues, it seems clear also that these changes are the result of the authors' trying to address (unsuccessfully) the various criticisms that have been presented against the PB principle. Of course, the fact that authors change their minds, clarify their claims, or reformulate their arguments is in no way a problem. After all, that is what we should expect of scholarly engagement and dialogue. Nonetheless, rather than recognizing the problems present in the original defense of the principle that forced them to rework several of the initial claims, the authors simply have insisted that many of those who have rejected PB have done so "because they are not clear about its precise content, grounds, or implications" (Savulescu and Kahane 2009, 276). Given the many ambiguities and inconsistencies present in the defense of this principle, critics could certainly be forgiven for "not being clear" about what exactly it involves and what its implications are.

In what follows, I take the 2009 version of the PB principle to be the relevant one; I am assuming that the authors believe it to be a more appropriate formulation. I argue that this refined version, and its defense, continue to be plagued by fatal problems. First, I will show that there are no good reasons to believe that a moral obligation to select the best child exists. Second, I will show that even if one were to grant its existence, this putative obligation fails to provide a guide for action. Finally, I will contend that even if one were to concede that the moral obligation in question can appropriately provide some direction to prospective parents, acceptance of such a duty has consequences that call into question its acceptability.

Selecting the Best Child One Can Have: Not a Moral Obligation

Two interrelated concerns can be raised regarding the existence of a moral obligation to select the best child parents can have. One relates to the appropriate grounds for such an obligation and the other to the force of the moral obligation. I first argue that there are no reasonable grounds for this duty. Second, I show that by the authors' own account, the obligation to select the best child has no moral force because it fails to present anyone with a moral demand.

At first sight, PB seems an implausible principle; after all, it entails that prospective parents must use a variety of invasive technologies to fulfill their moral obligations. Nonetheless, Savulescu and colleagues argue that the principle is well grounded. Some of their claims indicate that they take PB to be grounded on rationality. For instance, in his initial defense of the principle, Savulescu (2001b, 415) argued that morality "requires us to do what we have most reason to do."[1] Similarly, in their 2009 article, Savulescu and Kahane indicated that "general constraints on rationality instruct us to aim to have the most advantaged child" (282). For them, insofar as no other reason against selection exists, a person who has a good reason to have the best child is morally required to do so. Thus, given that parents care about the well-being of their children and that genetic factors affect well-being, unless they have a countervailing reason, prospective parents are said to have a reason to select the best child they can have on pain of irrationality.

But does morality require that we do what we have most reason to do? On its face, this claim seems implausible (Hotke 2014; Urbanek 2013). For example, I might have most reason to travel to Rome rather than Paris (e.g., the airline ticket to Rome is cheaper, the gelato is better, it is sunnier and I love warm weather), but it is certainly not the case that morality requires me to do so. Arguably, it might be the case that I would be irrational if, in spite of the fact that I believe I have most reason to go to Rome, I nonetheless chose to go to Paris, but it is clearly not the case that I would be acting immorally in making that choice.

---

1. Notice that "what one has most reason to do" can have different interpretations. For instance, it can be understood as "what one has in fact most reason to do" or as "what one believes one has most reason to do." Either way, this does not affect the argument presented here against Savulescu. Nonetheless, the difference is relevant in order to determine whether someone has done what Savulescu takes to be morally required.

Although it might be true that it is never irrational to be moral, this does not mean that it is always immoral to be irrational.

Perhaps the moral obligation to select the best child can be grounded on the more general duty parents have to care about the welfare of their children. Some of the discussion by Savulescu and Kahane (2009) seems to suggest that they have something like this in mind. They argue, for instance, that commonsense morality accepts that there is a moral defect in parents who intend to conceive a child but who nonetheless are indifferent as to whether the child in question will be born with the potential for a good life (Savulescu and Kahane 2009, 276). They also contend that commonsense morality leads many to agree that a couple would have reasons to wait if, because of some medical condition, they could have either a child with average health and talents now or an especially healthy and gifted child if they waited 1 month. By waiting, they say, these parents would be selecting a child who will have a better life (Savulescu and Kahane 2009, 276). For Savulescu and Kahane, these common practices and intuitions are simply an indication that it is implicit in commonsense morality that it is "often expected of parents to take the means to select future children with greater potential for well-being" (Savulescu and Kahane 2009, 277).

Let us put aside the fact that the authors offer no justification for why we should defer to commonsense morality in this respect. More importantly, it is not at all clear that commonsense morality entails implicitly or explicitly, parents' moral obligation to select a child who will have greater well-being. Certainly, one can accept that prospective parents have good reasons to care for the well-being of their children and also that genes play a role in human well-being. But without more assumptions that do not seem part of commonsense morality, it is not at all obvious that this entails that parents also "have reason to *aim* to have children who are more advantaged rather than leave this to chance or nature" (p. 276, emphasis in original). Caring about the well-being of one's children in no way entails that one ought to maximize their well-being. I care for my child's welfare, but doing so does not mean that I ought to take her to see the movie she wants rather than the one I prefer to see. Acceptance of a parental duty to care about the well-being of one's children involves, at most, agreement that using technologies such as in vitro fertilization (IVF) and preimplantation genetic diagnosis (PGD) could be *one way* to fulfill the general duty to care for one's children's welfare but not that using such technologies to select the best child is a moral obligation.

But perhaps this is all that PB calls for: Rather than a moral obligation, PB presents prospective parents with a moral reason to select the best child they can have. There is again at least some evidence supporting this reading. First, as we have seen, the reformulated principle of PB states that reproducers have a *significant moral reason* to act in a particular way—that is, to select the best child among the possible children they could have. Second, Savulescu and Kahane state that "selection of a future child is *morally permissible* and that parents *have reasons* to care about the potential well-being of future children" (Savulescu and Kahane 2009, 279, my emphasis). This is consistent with understanding PB as offering a moral reason rather than presenting prospective parents with a moral obligation. However, if this were all, PB would not be particularly controversial (Sparrow 2007). It seems trivial to say that prospective parents have some moral reason to choose characteristics, including genetic ones, that are likely to increase their children's well-being. If PB is understood in this way, it might be said to be grounded on the more general obligation that parents have to care about the welfare of their children, but in that case the principle seems unnecessary.

Nonetheless, a variety of claims made by these authors in their defense of PB calls this interpretation of the principle into question. First, the title of Savulescu and Kahane's (2009) article is "*The Moral Obligation* to Create Children with the Best Chance of the Best Life" (my emphasis). It would seem strange to use such a title if what the authors were planning to defend was a significantly less demanding claim. Second, at various points, these authors insist that PB involves a moral obligation. In their 2009 article, Savulescu and Kahane explicitly state, "[W]e present PB as a moral obligation" (277). In the initial article defending PB, Savulescu also explicitly talks about PB as involving a moral obligation and states that "we have *a moral obligation* to test for genetic contribution to non-disease states such as intelligence and to use this information in reproductive decision-making" (Savulescu 2001b, 414, my emphasis). Third, in both articles, the authors contend that egregious procreative choices deserve our moral disapproval, even if they do not call for legal punishment. Moral disapproval is an appropriate response when people fail to do what they are morally required to do but not when people are morally permitted to act or not in a particular way. Fourth, they claim that PB requires prospective parents to select the best child unless doing so is likely to lead to a very significant loss of well-being for existing people. PB, they say, imposes a reason that cannot be dismissed lightly. As they insist:

> When the *obligation* to have the most advantaged child is not overridden by sufficiently strong opposing moral reasons, it will be true that parents ought, all things considered, to select the most advantaged child. PB is not just the claim that parents are permitted to choose the most advantaged child. If the competing reasons are stronger, then it is not permissible to choose the most advantaged child. And if there aren't such reasons, or they are weaker, then *it is not morally permissible* to choose anything less than the best (Savulescu and Kahane 2009, 278, my emphasis).

Given this evidence, it is difficult to understand PB as a moral recommendation rather than a moral demand. But perhaps the ambiguities and inconsistencies in their claims can be explained by the fact that the authors conflate moral reasons and moral obligations (Sparrow 2007). Indeed, there is some evidence that supports this possibility. For instance, in their 2009 article, Savulescu and Kahane explicitly state:

> Those who prefer to think of such reasons as generated by moral obligations should also think of reasons of PB as generated by an obligation. Since we do not think that anything turns on this distinction, in what follows we will use moral reason and moral obligation interchangeably (278).

This is a peculiar position, to say the least. It seems that moral reasons might recommend a particular act, and they might also outweigh reasons for acting otherwise, without it necessarily being the case that the action in question is morally required (Darwall 2010). For example, if my friend has a cold and she would like to have my company, the fact that she wants my company gives me a moral reason to go to see her. It might even give me a reason that outweighs other reasons for not going, such as preferring to watch a new television program I have been excitedly waiting for. But this hardly shows that I have a moral obligation to go visit my friend. Certainly, moral obligations are usually understood as moral reasons. But it is not the case that just any moral reason can be thought of as a moral obligation. Arguably, obligations are moral reasons of a special kind. They present us with a moral demand for which we are legitimately answerable. Indeed, if a person fails to do what she is morally obligated to do, she does something wrong, and if she lacks a valid excuse, she is thought to be blameworthy. However, if a person fails to do what she has a moral reason to do, she need not be considered to have done anything wrong. Thus, if I decide against visiting my friend because I expect my mother to call me that day, because I need to do some work, or because the weather is unpleasant, it seems that I have done nothing morally wrong. If, on the other hand, I have promised my friend that I will visit her, none of those reasons would justify my breaking the promise, and I would indeed be doing something morally wrong if I failed to visit her. Moreover, I would be blameworthy.

It appears that Savulescu and Kahane are concerned that taking moral obligations to be something different from moral reasons commits one to seeing moral obligations as absolute. Thus they say: "Some hold that if there is a moral obligation to do X, then this implies that we absolutely must do X."[2] And they continue:

> It is doubtful that any non-trivial moral principle is this strong. PB is not an absolute obligation. It is the claim that there is a *significant moral reason* to choose the better child. The principle states, not what people invariably must do, but what they have significant moral reason to do.

But this is absurd. Savulescu and Kahane's claims to the contrary, conceptualizing moral obligations as having more strength than just any moral reason in no way commits one to taking them to be absolute. Clearly, one can defend the idea that moral obligations, although reasons of a special, weighty kind, are nonetheless defeasible. That is, they can be pro tanto obligations. They are, however, not defeasible by just any other reason, indeed not even by just any other *moral* reason. My promise to visit my friend might be defeated by the proverbial stranger in need of

2. Indeed the authors claim, mistakenly, that I hold such a view (Savulescu and Kahane 2009, 278, note 17).

urgent help but arguably not by any of the reasons I mentioned earlier. Indeed, some have argued that even in cases in which one is justified in acting contrary to a moral obligation, there is still some residual obligation (e.g. Williams 1965; Marcus 1980). Thus, even if my promise to visit my friend is overridden by my obligation to help a stranger in dire need, my promise has not been voided, and I am still required to do something about it, such as give an explanation to my friend. Moreover, moral obligations that justifiably fail to be fulfilled call for certain moral emotions, such as regret (Strawson 1962). But none of this seems to be the case when one simply fails to do what one has some moral reason to do. If this is correct, much indeed seems to turn on the distinction between moral reasons and moral obligations. They cannot be treated as equivalent, not at least without providing an appropriate defense for such a stance, which the authors fail to do.

Let us summarize the arguments so far. I have argued that PB presents us with either a moral obligation or a moral recommendation about a way for prospective parents to care for the welfare of their children. I have shown that Savulescu and Kahane have offered no appropriate grounds for PB as a moral obligation. Thus, PB can indeed present prospective parents with a reason to select. However, if it is understood as simply offering a recommendation, PB seems trivial and unnecessary.

But Savulescu and colleagues cannot establish that there is an obligation to select the best child, and not only because they have failed to provide grounds for PB. They also fail to show that there is such a moral obligation because, by their own account, the principle has no moral force. Let us see why. Even if we grant that PB presents prospective parents with a pro tanto obligation that is defeasible, that obligation can be defeated only by stronger pro tanto obligations. For instance, if the obligation to select the best child conflicts with the obligation parents have to existent children, then PB might be defeated. What reasons do Savulescu and Kahane take to be sufficiently strong to possibly defeat PB? It is not completely clear. They indicate that reasons related to the welfare of the parents, or of existing children or others, as well as possible harm to others, could defeat the putative moral obligation to select the best child (Savulescu and Kahane 2009, 278). This is scarcely helpful in determining when PB must be followed. All kinds of activities, significant and insignificant, can be thought to affect people's welfare, and we saw in chapter 3 that determining what constitutes harm depends on a variety of normative assumptions. Thus, not all reasons related to the welfare of parents, existing children, or other human beings would be strong enough to defeat a pro tanto obligation to select the best child. For instance, if the prospective parents would rather use the money required for IVF and PGD for a summer trip, such a decision would hardly constitute a consideration against PB even though it is related to the parents' welfare. Similarly, if a couple's children would be upset by the fact that they were conceived without the use of reprogenetic technologies and would rather have a sibling similarly conceived, that would scarcely count as a weighty reason against using PB even though it pertains to the welfare of existent children. Nonetheless, one could interpret such reasons in a way that is consistent with PB as a pro tanto moral obligation. For example, if use of selective technologies would ruin parents financially, then their own welfare and that of their existent children might be thought to provide a sufficiently strong reason to defeat PB. Likewise, if serious harms to society could be shown to result from reprogenetic technologies, this would also constitute a reason against PB.

More problematic, however, is the authors' contention that considerations such as prospective parents' stands on moral questions about genetic manipulation, the use of IVF, abortion, or the moral status of embryos are deemed legitimate reasons to defeat their obligation to select the best child (Savulescu and Kahane 2009, 278). This is certainly peculiar. What one's stands are on all of these issues is inextricably tied to the moral obligation in question. That is, PB demands the use of IVF and PGD; it calls for the genetic manipulation of embryos by PGD; and it mandates the creation and destruction of embryos so as to be able to select the best one. Hence, arguing that one's stands on genetic manipulation, IVF, abortion, or the moral status of embryos count as legitimate reasons against PB is arguing that one has a moral obligation to select the best child unless one morally opposes embryo selection. It would be like claiming that people have a moral obligation to limit their contribution to climate change and then indicate that the scope of that obligation depends on one's moral stand on the use of public transportation or recycling, beliefs about the moral status of future generations, or attitudes toward distant people. In other words, people have a moral obligation to limit their contribution to climate change unless they happen to have beliefs that conflict with caring about the causes and effects of climate change.

Claiming that one's stands about issues that are intrinsic to the discharging of a duty to select are relevant to fulfilling such a duty involves a further problem. PB would apply only to those who hold particular moral beliefs about embryos, IVF, or PGD; that is, it would apply only to those whose moral beliefs are consistent with the moral permissibility of abortion and the use of IVF and PGD, but it would not apply to those whose moral beliefs conflict with the moral permissibility of these activities. This makes PB a very strange moral duty indeed. Of course, sometimes people's moral duties conflict, and they have to determine which obligations to discharge when it is not possible to discharge all of them. But Savulescu and Kahane's claims leave people who have particular moral stands completely off the hook. Indeed, no conflict of duties would exist for these individuals because it is built into the understanding of this moral obligation that if one's stands are inconsistent with fulfilling it, it can legitimately be ignored. It is true also that some moral obligations apply only to some people and not to others. Role obligations, the sorts of obligations we have by virtue of occupying a particular social role, apply only to some individuals (i.e., those occupying the relevant role, such as a parent, professor, or daughter) but not to others. Clearly, for instance, PB applies only to prospective parents and not to those who have no wish to become parents. But PB conceived in this way would place a moral demand on some prospective parents (i.e., those who have the appropriate stands about genetic manipulation, IVF, PGD, and the status of embryos) but not on other prospective parents, those who simply reject the stands called for by PB.

The authors do seem to accept that PB has a very limited scope (Savulescu and Kahane, 2009, 278). Nonetheless, they insist that this does not justify an outright denial of the principle. However, their assertion is incorrect. If PB is understood as presenting prospective parents with a pro tanto moral demand and yet can be circumscribed by moral considerations that are intrinsic to the demand in question, this does show that the principle is false—that is, it cannot constitute a moral obligation to select the best child. To argue that in this case PB would still be true is simply to misunderstand what moral obligations entail.

Procreative Beneficence: Failing to Guide Action

Whatever other roles moral principles may have, telling people what actions are right and wrong is certainly one of them. Moral principles are arguably in the business of helping to guide conduct, of providing direction to agents about what decisions to make or what to do. This need not imply that principles offer a decision-making procedure that will always guide agents to do the right thing or that require no judgment. But if a moral principle cannot, with some reliability, guide people's decisions and actions, that would seem to call into question not just the usability of the principle but also its value. So, how useful is PB in guiding prospective parents' decisions and actions, in helping them do the right thing and select the best child that they can have? Arguably, at least when dealing with traits not related to diseases, it is not very useful at all. This is so for several reasons. First, it is difficult to determine when the principle obtains. Clearly, PB places demands on individuals who have decided to have a child.[3] But when are prospective parents obligated to discharge their duty to select? Is it at the moment they are trying to conceive? Is it when they realize they have a desire to become parents, even if they are not planning to do so in the near future? Clearly, these two possible alternatives make the set of people to whom PB applies narrower or broader, respectively. Moreover, it is not just the set of people to whom PB applies but also the range of actions to which the principle applies that is significantly different depending on when prospective parents are obligated to fulfill their duties. If PB applies to people who are actively seeking to have a child, then it seems to ask of them that they use reprogenetic technologies instead of the usual means of reproduction because coital reproduction does not allow for comparison and selection among candidate children. Still, imagine that the set of embryos available at a particular point fails to be the best that the prospective parents could have. Suppose, for instance, that

---

3. This is an improvement over the initial formulation of PB, which could be interpreted as requiring people both to have children and to select the best one they could have. In its second formulation, individuals with no interest in having children are not subject to PB.

all of the available embryos seem to have inherited a mutation from one of the progenitors that increases the probability that the child produced will be shy. Are these prospective parents morally obligated to try IVF again in order to obtain a new set of embryos that might include some without the mutation in question, given that such is possible? Or is this a trait whose effect on well-being is not important enough to outweigh the costs and health risks to a woman using IVF? And if it is not, would any non–disease-related traits be significant enough to call for the use of reprogenetic technologies? It is true that the PB principle permits parents to select a child that is less than the best if such is the only option, but it says nothing about what the relevant comparison set is. Is it only the one composed of the embryos obtained after a single IVF cycle, or does PB demand that prospective parents try more than one IVF cycle if they believe they could achieve a better set of embryos?

If, on the other hand, PB is relevant not just to prospective parents who are actively trying to have a child but to anyone who has the desire to become a parent, even if not in the immediate future, then it would seem to call for these individuals to consider the many ways in which their choices are likely to affect the children they can have in the future. This involves, of course, not only choices about what partner to select (Urbanek 2013) but also decisions about what university to attend, what to study, what job to accept, and where to live. Even if Savulescu and Kahane want to claim that PB does not require prospective parents to give up personal projects, it is difficult to see how PB would not call for them to consider the ways in which their choices are likely to affect their future children's well-being and to act accordingly. After all, Savulescu and Kahane (2009, 283) insist that "reasons of PB are continuous with familiar parental duties governing the spacing of our children and the circumstances under which we should have them."

A second reason to question the usefulness of PB in guiding action is related to the difficulty of determining what is meant by the caveat "and selection is possible" in the principle's formulation. Does it mean insofar as the technologies to select the best embryos exist? If one has the financial means to use such technologies? As long as a variety of embryos exist? If there is more than one partner, school, job, or city available from which to choose? As before, the exact meaning of this caveat will have very different implications for guiding action. If it is a technical requirement, then the caveat seems unnecessary because the technologies do, in fact, exist. If it refers to financial possibilities, then when does the constraint apply? It would seem that those who are poor would clearly be exempt from the demands of PB, but what about those who have the financial means but only if they give up on other things?

Third, PB calls for prospective parents to select the best or most advantaged child that they can have. Determining what counts as the best or most advantaged child is not an easy task (de Melo-Martin 2004; Parker 2007). Savulescu and Kahane (2009, 279) contend that PB is compatible with several theories of well-being including hedonism, desire-fulfillment accounts, and objective list theories. They seem to think that this speaks in favor of PB, but it is not clear that it does. As Sparrow (2007) pointed out, the PB principle, on any of these accounts, will turn out to have either counterintuitive or incoherent results. For instance, prospective parents who have a hedonistic conception of well-being would act appropriately were they to care exclusively about choosing the child whose brain chemistry is more likely to cause the feeling of pleasure—and indeed, they would be obligated to choose such an action if it were an option. Similarly, on a desire-fulfillment account, parents would have reasons to select children who would grow up to have less ambition or curiosity because they would be more likely to have easily satisfied preferences and thus would have better lives.

More importantly for the ability of PB to guide action is the difficulty in comparing characteristics that are more or less likely to make one life go better than another (de Melo-Martin, 2004; Parker 2007; Hauskeller 2013). For instance, imagine parents having to decide which of three embryos is likely to result in the child who is expected to have the best life: embryo A shows a predisposition to asthma, has gene variants for above-average memory and intelligence, has a predisposition for physical strength, is likely to be short, and has blue eyes; embryo B is likely to be taller, with high endurance, average intelligence, physical beauty, and brown eyes; and embryo C is likely to have average height, good memory, a sunny attitude, perfect pitch, and a proneness to stress.[4] Of course, we can make the scenario as complicated as we wish. Indeed, prospective parents are more likely to face complicated scenarios rather than simpler ones such as those described by proponents. So given the likely complexities, what are good prospective parents to do if they want to act according to the demands of the PB principle? It is difficult to see how PB could be of any help in guiding parental decisions in these and similar cases.

Savulescu and Kahane have tried to respond to this criticism in several ways. For example, they have argued that this

---

4. A reminder here is in order. As I indicated in chapter 1, engaging with proponents of reprogenetics can prove tricky if one takes scientific and technological knowledge seriously. On the one hand, there are no reasons to believe that genetic testing will ever provide anyone with reliable information about most—or any—of these traits. On the other hand, given that proponents of reprogenetics seem to have an unwavering faith in the power of genetic testing (and genetic enhancement), and given that they often use these unlikely scenarios to make their case, it seems appropriate to consider them so as to evaluate their implications. Thus, I use the examples here simply to make my case, not because I believe that they have any plausibility.

objection presupposes the belief that there is no such thing as a better or best life (Savulescu and Kahane 2009, 279). But there are various problems with this response. First, the notions of a "better" and a "best" life are not equivalent. One can agree that, all things being equal, a life that does not contain toothaches is *better* than one that does, but that hardly means that a life without toothaches is *the best* life. Second, pointing out the difficulty for parents in scenarios such as the one described is perfectly consistent with having particular beliefs about whether one life is better than another. What calling attention to the difficulties that prospective parents are likely to face when discharging their moral duty does is simply to point out that what makes a life better or worse is a complex matter and that PB is unlikely to be very helpful in guiding prospective parents' decisions.

Savulescu and Kahane have also attempted to respond to this criticism by claiming that common morality already asks prospective parents to make such complex choices and that PB is simply an extension of those types of decisions. This is, however, far from obvious. First, as already indicated, common morality does not require prospective parents to maximize their children's well-being; it requires that they care about it. Second, when prospective parents make decisions that are likely to affect their children's welfare, such decisions are of the form, "this is likely to make the life of my child better." That is, the comparison is between the life of the child if one does A or if one does B (e.g., if one sends the child to school A or to school B). In ordinary life, parents are not required to choose between child A and child B according to which one is more likely to have the best life.

Savulescu and Kahane have also argued that in complex cases where different forms of life might be equally good or contain incomparable forms of well-being, prospective parents following PB are free to choose any of the available options. But, at least in the case of non-disease characteristics,[5] it is hard to imagine a context in which prospective parents will not find themselves in the situation of being able to choose any of the available choices. After all, people with all kinds of physical, psychological, and character traits can have comparably good lives.

Finally, Savulescu and Kahane have also maintained that concerns about parents' choices are not really concerns about the truth of PB but about its misapplication. This is also incorrect. The issue at stake is not that parents could make the wrong choices because they are misapplying PB.[6] The concern is that PB offers prospective parents little assistance in deciding what they should choose. That these difficulties do not need to render PB false (Hotke 2014) might well be the case, but it is also irrelevant. The point is whether PB can help guide prospective parents' decisions. The PB principle makes those decisions often impossible and usually very difficult, and this is arguably a good reason to reject it.

Negative Consequences of Procreative Beneficence

Also counting against PB are the negative consequences that would follow from a commitment to it. These adverse consequences would affect both individuals who take their moral obligations seriously and society as a whole. What are these negative consequences? As we have seen, insofar as the PB principle is thought to have any strength, it is excessively demanding. Even

5. I am not suggesting that this would not be the case also when dealing with many diseases and disabilities. Indeed, I believe that in such cases prospective parents would also have good reasons to choose a variety of alternative options.

6. In fact, it does not seem that PB could exclude many choices as wrong, given that the principle is compatible with all major theories of well-being and with various conceptions of the good life.

if we limit its application to those who are actively seeking to have a child, PB calls for prospective parents to use IVF and PGD. In countries like the United States, where the use of these technologies depends on ability to pay, this would mean significant financial burdens for many prospective parents.[7] Proposing that these technologies be available to all prospective parents is not simply unrealistic but also problematic given the opportunity costs of the use of these technologies.

As we have seen, Savulescu and colleagues might object that PB does not present prospective parents with an absolute moral obligation but with a pro tanto one. Nonetheless, as indicated, this hardly solves the problem. Not just any reason can outweigh a pro tanto moral obligation. Even if we were to take financial burdens as sufficient to outweigh the moral obligation to select, this does not solve the problematic implications of PB. First, as is well known, many parents go to great lengths to ensure the well-being of their children. And they do so even when there is not a moral obligation making such demands. Thus, and insofar as we believe that people ought to take their moral obligations seriously, it is likely that many prospective parents will want to fulfill their duty to select the best child even at great cost to themselves. Second, even if those who are unable to discharge their obligation to use IVF and PGD for financial reasons are thought to be excused from doing so, this does not eliminate the undesirable implications of PB for individual parents. When people are regularly excused from doing what we would consider wrong, in this case not selecting for the best child, they are consigned to a moral underclass of individuals who, because of their economic situation, are incapable of behaving morally.

---

7. Of note, the use of IVF also involves significant physical burdens for women, but because chapter 6 deals specifically with the neglect of women in discussions of reprogenetics, I do not discuss here burdens that affect women in particular.

Furthermore, feelings of regret and guilt are common, and arguably appropriate, even when one is justified in not fulfilling a particular moral duty. Given the fact that most parents would want to do as much as they could to improve the conditions of their children's lives, most of them, if aware of their moral obligation to select for the best child but unable to do so, would likely experience regret and remorse because of their inability to do what is morally right. Additionally, because it is difficult in many cases to know whether people's failure to meet this parental obligation is justified, individuals are likely to be morally condemned. Undeniably, the fact that people might feel remorse or regret for failing to discharge their moral duties is not a reason to reject a moral obligation. But the fact that a moral obligation to use reprogenetics could not be fulfilled by the majority of the population seems a good reason to question its validity.

Following the PB mandate has negative implications not just for individual parents but also for society in general (de Melo-Martin 2004; Sparrow 2007). First, the effects of many different prospective parents' fulfilling their moral obligation to select the best child could sometimes lead to self-defeating outcomes. Many of the traits selected would be chosen both because they are valued in our society and because they offer those who have them a competitive advantage. Take, for instance, height. In societies that value stature, there would be good reason to believe that being tall would favorably impact a child's well-being. It is true that selection does not allow parents to make their children taller than a given range (i.e., they are limited by their own genetic endowment). Nonetheless, if a couple select for such a trait in their child but nobody else does, then the selected embryo will be better off (all other things being equal). However, if all prospective parents are making the same choice with respect to height, then the degree of variation would presumably remain unchanged. Thus, the prospective parents' selection would be self-defeating. Given the costs, health risks, and time involved in the selection of children, it would seem quite problematic to not simply allow but morally require prospective parents to select for traits when the effects on the well-being of the children chosen will be nonexistent. Granted, this problem of aggregate effects will appear mostly in cases of selection for non–disease-related genes that offer some competitive advantage in the society in which one lives. Such a self-defeating effect would not occur when selecting for traits that might be good for individuals to have even if everyone else has them too (e.g., intelligence).[8] Nonetheless, arguably, the great majority of traits for which parents can conceivably select are unlikely to be of this type.

Second, in an unjust world like ours, where certain physical and psychological traits are particularly valued and others are devalued, parents trying to select for the best child they can have are likely to choose in ways that will contribute to and increase social injustice. In sexist, racist, and homophobic societies, PB would require of parents that they select children who are boys, as fair-skinned as possible, and heterosexual. And insofar as PB requires that prospective parents choose their partners according to characteristics that are likely to contribute to their future children's well-being, it would call for both white and black people in a racist society to try to have children only with white people, because fairer-skinned children will be expected to have better lives. In societies that value particular traits such as height, strength, beauty, self-control, ambition, or high memory, PB would require of parents that they select the embryos most likely to conform to those characteristics. It is true that for many of these traits there are no reasons to believe that genetic

8. "Intelligence" is not a univocal concept, so much will depend on how it is conceptualized.

testing will give us reliable predictions, but for some of them (e.g., sex), it will.[9] In any case, that application of the obligation to select can plausibly contribute to social injustice is certainly a reason against it. This reason is even weightier when one considers the fact that, according to Savulescu, prospective parents have reasons to follow PB even if selection for the traits in question increases injustice and affects the child's well-being only minimally.

Savulescu and colleagues have attempted to deal with this problematic consequence in various ways. For instance, Savulescu has denied that social injustice could result from the use of PB. According to him, insofar as selection of particular traits contributes to inequality, it is unlikely that such traits would promote well-being (Savulescu 2001b, 424). But this claim is either true but irrelevant or simply false. It is irrelevant because prospective parents following the PB principle might be unaware of how their decisions contribute to their communities. It might well be the case that in a sexist society where parents systematically select for boys, the well-being of those boys might diminish because of the effects in society of fewer females. But parents would realize this only after the choices contributing to injustice have been made. Furthermore, the claim might simply be false. If, as is currently the case in many places, access to reprogenetic technologies depends on ability to pay, those who have the financial means will select for children who have the most valued traits in a particular society, whereas the rest will have to rely on chance. It is quite

9. Of course, that genetic testing is unlikely to give reliable prediction about many of these trains is a response that Savulescu and other proponents of reprogenetic technologies cannot give. After all, they would welcome the development of biomedical knowledge so that genetic testing is able to reliably predict these non-disease traits. Moreover, their contention is that increases in social injustice need not count as a reason against fulfilling one's obligation to select the best child.

likely that the well-being of these selected children would not be diminished while at the same time their parents' choices would have contributed to the increases in social inequality. After all, many of the non-disease traits that parents would select for in a particular social context are likely to be selected because they give a competitive advantage to their possessor. Similarly, in racist societies, it is implausible that the selection of fair-skinned children would ever contribute to either a decrease in well-being for fair-skinned selected children or a decrease in social injustices against those with darker skin (Sparrow 2007).

Savulescu and Kahane have also tried to address these negative consequences by conceding that for some parents, concern for social justice might outweigh their pro tanto reason to select the best child. But this is only a matter of personal choice. In any case, the moral requirement to select the best child means that people are morally justified in selecting for traits that might improve their child's well-being slightly, even if doing so results in social injustice.

If the arguments presented here are correct, and I believe they are, PB has nothing going for it. To the extent that the principle is understood as simply offering some reason to prospective parents, it seems trivial and unnecessary. If, on the other hand, PB is taken to present prospective parents with a moral obligation—a pro tanto moral obligation but a moral obligation nonetheless—its proponents have offered no plausible grounding for it. Furthermore, by their own account, PB seems to be a peculiar moral obligation, one that appears to make no demands on any prospective parents who have any reason whatsoever to reject it. Additionally, PB seems to be useless in guiding action. Finally, a commitment to PB would likely have significant negative consequences, not only for particular individuals but for society in general.

The Moral Obligation to Enhance our Offspring

Proponents of reprogenetics have not only argued that prospective parents have a moral obligation to *select* the best child they can have, but they have also defended a moral obligation to *enhance* one's future children. It should be clear that grounding this putative moral duty on the duty parents have to care for their children is even more implausible than using such grounds to defend a duty to select the best child. This is so because a moral obligation to enhance entails not only that parents must use IVF and PGD in order to select one of the embryos thus created but also that they must use reprogenetic technologies to modify those embryos' genetic endowments.

Likewise, an obligation to enhance would be scarcely useful in guiding action. Indeed, action-guiding problems would only increase, given the difficulties in determining what constitutes an enhancement. For instance, Harris (2007, 2) claims that enhancements are those things that "make us better at doing some of the things we want to do, better at experiencing the world through all of our senses, better at assimilating and processing what we experience, better at remembering and understanding things, stronger, more competent, more of everything we want to be." According to this definition, it seems that only scientific and technological ignorance could limit what one must attempt to enhance in one's offspring. But insofar as the technological ability exists to ensure that embryos are manipulated so as to give them "more of everything," this definition offers little help to prospective parents who want to do the right thing and appropriately discharge their duties.

It should be clear that the negative consequences discussed earlier with regard to the effects on prospective parents' moral lives when they are unable to meet the obligation to select, as well as the adverse consequences for social justice, would be exacerbated by commitment to a moral obligation to enhance. Therefore, as in the case of PB, there are good reasons to call into question the moral obligation to enhance our offspring. However, the obligation to enhance is actually open to additional problems, for two reasons. First, proponents of reprogenetic technologies usually argue that the obligation to enhance is grounded on general harm prevention principles. Second, this moral obligation involves the manipulation of embryos and not just their selection. I discuss these concerns in the following sections.

The Obligation to Enhance as Harm Prevention

Both Harris and Savulescu have argued that the moral obligation to enhance simply follows from our general obligation to prevent harm. For Harris (2007, 58) "the overwhelming medical imperative for both therapy and enhancement is to prevent harm and confer benefit." For both authors, failing to confer benefits is equivalent to harming the individual. Thus, Savulescu (2005) insists:

> Once technology affords us with the power to enhance our and our children's lives, to fail to do so will be to be responsible for the consequences. To fail to treat our children's disease is to harm them. To fail to prevent them getting depression is to harm them. To fail to improve their physical, musical, psychological and other capacities is to harm them, just as it would be to harm them if we gave them a toxic substance that stunted or reduced these capacities" (38).

Likewise, Harris sees harms and benefits as a continuum, so that the reasons we might have to prevent harm to others are continuous with the reasons we have to provide a benefit to them.

For him, "to decide to withhold a benefit is in a sense to harm the individual we decline to benefit. We have reasons for declining to create or confer even trivial harms, and we have reasons to confer and not withhold even small benefits" (Harris 2001, 386). This is, however, implausible. It is not generally the case that failing to confer a benefit always counts as a harm—or at least, insofar as it does count as a harm, that it is morally wrong to do so. Thus, it would be a benefit to me if Warren Buffet were to offer me a fully paid vacation to Rome, but it is implausible to say that his failure to do so harms me in the relevant moral sense. It is even more implausible to say that he has done something morally wrong. Indeed, a theory that equates failing to benefit with harming would be so demanding that it is unlikely anyone could ever behave morally. This does not mean that all cases of causing harm are always worse than all cases of preventing harm or failing to benefit. But it does call into question the claim that failing to benefit is always a moral wrong and that benefiting is thus a moral obligation. Of course, we could agree that we have *some* reasons to confer and not withhold benefits, but those reasons would seem to be easily defeasible and thus hardly the kinds of reasons that amount to a moral obligation.

Arguing that failing to benefit is equivalent to harming—and is therefore morally wrong—is also inconsistent with these authors' position on the non-identity problem. As mentioned in chapter 3, the non-identity problem, discussed most famously by Derek Parfit (1984), calls attention to the difficulty of accounting for the apparent wrongness of some actions that affect who is born. Consider the following case. Because she is suffering from an infection that can affect a fetus, if a woman decides to have a child now, the child will be born with certain disease, but if she waits a few weeks, the child who is born will not suffer from that disease. She decides to have the child now. The non-identity problem calls attention to the fact that even if her actions appear to make things worse for the child brought into existence, it is not clear that she has committed a wrong. Had she chosen otherwise, the future child would not have been the same person, but a non-identical child instead. Therefore, it is not obvious that what she has done is bad for the child who is born, who will have a worthwhile life.

The non-identity problem has led to a voluminous amount of literature offering solutions to it (see, for instance, Boonin 2014; Brock 1995; Harman 2004; Roberts and Wasserman 2009). Savulescu and Harris have taken the non-identity problem to show that concerns about the welfare of the child in reproductive cases have little force.[10] For instance, when defending sex selection practices, Savulescu (1999) writes:

> Most importantly, without sex selection, without a unique sperm and egg uniting, that particular child would not have existed. Even if the child is disadvantaged psychologically, this is only wrong from the child's perspective if its life is so bad that it is not worth living (374).

Likewise, in an article defending egg freezing for social reasons, he argues:

> [E]ven if IVF of older women results in physical damage to the child produced, that child has not been harmed by being conceived by social IVF (except if its life is so bad that it is not worth living). If the couple had used another means of conception at a different time, a different child would have been born. This is the non-identity problem and it reduces much of

10. This does not mean that Harris and Savulescu think that the woman has done nothing wrong, but for them the wrongness of her action is explained in non–person-affecting terms and thus is not grounded on the fact that the child's welfare has presumably been negatively affected.

the force of the so called "child welfare" arguments against reproductive technologies, including social IVF (Goold and Savulescu 2009, 55).

Harris has been equally explicit concerning the difficulty of using arguments about a child's well-being as reasons to reject reprogenetic technologies. For example, in his defense of reproductive cloning, he rejects a variety of objections to the practice that are based on the welfare of the child brought about by cloning and concludes as follows:

> [W]here we judge the circumstances of a future person to be less than ideal but not so bad as to deprive that individual of a worthwhile existence, then we lack the moral justification to impose our ideals on others. The difference we are looking for is the difference between considerations which would clearly blight the life of the resulting child, and consideration that would merely make existence suboptimal in some sense (Burley and Harris 1999, 113).

And in his spirited defense of sex selection, he argues:

> [C]omplaints that parents who would use gender selection are attempting to shape or mold their child are simply incoherent. They may of course be choosing what sorts of children will come into existence, but none of those children have any legitimate or even coherent complaint, for they could not have had an alternative life free of such externally imposed choices" (Harris 2007, 159).

Now, if these cases indicate that the child who is born has not been harmed in the relevant moral sense, then, even if we were to accept the implausible view that failing to enhance our future children is tantamount to harming them, it does not seem that the children in question will have motive for complaint. Granted, Savulescu and Harris could claim that cases of enhancement fail to be non-identity cases. However, this is true only under a conception of identity that is tied to a particular egg and sperm. But we can question such a notion of identity. It might well be that some enhanced characteristics are unlikely to affect a person's identity (e.g., being a couple of inches taller). But at least some enhancements defended by Harris and Savulescu (e.g., self-control, certain cognitive abilities, radical life extension) are plausibly understood as identity-transforming. If this is so, then their take on the non-identity problem seems to prevent them from claiming that prospective parents have done something wrong by failing to enhance their future children.

Harris and Savulescu could still try to defend their claim that enhancements are a moral obligation while maintaining their position regarding the non-identity problem. They could argue that prospective parents who fail to enhance their future children have done something morally wrong because they have failed to benefit them but, because their failure to benefit their children does not amount to a serious and significant harm, the reproductive choices of such prospective parents ought not to be interfered with legally. This hardly solves the problem. After all, the non-identity problem concerns what we *morally* owe people, not what we have legal reasons to do. Moreover, their arguments regarding non-identity cases are not simply that we have no justification to interfere with people's reproductive choices but that the child has not been harmed.

Negative Consequences of a Duty to Enhance

If the negative consequences that arguably can follow from a duty to select the best child are worrisome, the ones resulting from a duty to enhance our offspring are even more so. This is the case because, whereas parents fulfilling the obligation to select have to content themselves with the genetic endowment their embryos have, enhancement technologies would allow parents to manipulate such endowment.

As we have already indicated, the reprogenetic technologies needed to enhance offspring are expensive, so access to them will be restricted to those with the ability to pay. Similarly, the traits likely to be enhanced are those that offer children a competitive advantage, even if that is not the goal. Thus, one might want to enhance a future child's memory, height, strength, and so on because one thinks that doing so would make the child's life better, but clearly those traits offer competitive advantages in many human societies. This choice, then, is likely to increase financial disparities and the effects that such disparities have on benefits such as political influence, access to education, and health care.

It is true, as proponents of reprogenetic technologies like to remind us, that unequal access to technological developments is a common occurrence in our societies. But this fact by itself is hardly a reason to disregard increases in inequality that arguably could result from the use of enhancement technologies. Even if equality is not valued for its own sake, there is good evidence that increases in inequality correlate with negative societal outcomes such as lower population health, higher crime rates, lower democratic participation, and erosion of public trust (Wilkinson and Pickett 2010). More importantly, insofar as the development and use of these technologies constitutes a moral obligation, as Harris and Savulescu would have it, the increase in unjust inequalities will actually be morally sanctioned. After all, prospective parents with the financial means to use these technologies in order to enhance their offspring would only be doing what is morally required.

But, as in the case of selection, social justice concerns are not limited to an increase in inequalities between those who will have access to reprogenetic technologies and those who will not. In sexist, racist, classist, ableist, and homophobic societies like ours, prospective parents will have reasons to enhance their offspring in ways that conform to sexist, racist, classist, ableist, and homophobic values. Whereas, with embryo selection, parents with darker skin, for instance, could at most attempt to select the embryo that is likely to produce the child with the lightest skin tone, enhancement technologies could be aimed at engineering such a trait. Similarly, parents who think their best child would be one who is heterosexual would not need to rely on genetic chance and could genetically intervene to ensure the sexual orientation of their future child. And here, also, it is not simply that prospective parents would be free to engineer their children according to their own prejudicial values. Prospective parents who find such values problematic might still feel pressured to ensure that their children will have better chances in an unjust world. This complicity with immoral values would again be cloaked under the claim that parents are simply doing what is morally required.

Simply pointing out that the obligation to enhance is a moral but not a legal obligation and thus that, provided they do not harm others, parents are free to enhance their children as they see fit but the state cannot coerce them, fails to address these concerns. First, insofar as one takes one's moral obligations seriously, one would want to discharge them. If so, a moral obligation to enhance provides parents with a very strong reason to do so, whether or not the state can compel them to act (Sparrow 2011). Even if some parents worry about increasing social injustice, they will have to weigh that concern against their obligation to their children. Moreover, some parents will surely not be particularly disturbed about engineering their children in ways that endorse and foster morally defective values. Second, as we have said, failing to discharge one's moral obligations requires justification. Thus, parents who choose not to be complicit with prejudicial values and decide against enhancing their children will be open to moral condemnation. Thus, when moral obligations are the issue, coercion by the state is not the only reason for concern.

Conclusion

Reprogenetic technologies can give prospective parents significant power over many of their future children's characteristics. These technologies now allow prospective parents to select embryos according to particular desired traits, and they might also give prospective parents the option to enhance certain characteristics. Although until now most of the uses of these technologies have been directed toward selection of embryos that are free of a variety of genetic mutations associated with diseases, they can also be used to select for genetic variants unrelated to disease. Proponents of reprogenetic technologies such as Harris and Savulescu have welcomed and embraced these possibilities. Their enthusiasm has led them not only to defend the moral permissibility of using these technologies for both disease-related and non–disease-related characteristics but also to espouse a moral obligation to select and enhance future offspring. In this chapter, I have argued that there are no reasons to accept that such obligations exist. Savulescu and Harris have failed to offer plausible grounds for a moral obligation to select or enhance future children. Moreover, even if the existence of these obligations were granted, their usefulness in guiding the decisions and actions of prospective parents leaves much to be desired. Finally, I have called attention to the negative consequences that are likely to follow from endorsing and fulfilling these putative moral obligations. Given all of these fatal problems, one wonders why proponents of these moral obligations continue supporting them so enthusiastically.

References

Bennett, R. 2009. The fallacy of the principle of procreative beneficence. *Bioethics* 23 (5):265–73.

Boonin, David. 2014. *The non-identity problem and the ethics of future people*. New York: Oxford University Press.

Brock, D. W. 1995. The nonidentity problem and genetic harms: the case of wrongful handicaps. *Bioethics* 9 (3–4):269–75.

Burley, J., and J. Harris. 1999. Human cloning and child welfare. *Journal of Medical Ethics* 25 (2):108–13.

Darwall, Stephen L. 2010. Moral obligation: form and substance. *Proceedings of the Aristotelian Society* 60 (Part 1):31–46.

de Melo-Martin, Inmaculada. 2004. On our obligation to select the best children: a reply to Savulescu. *Bioethics* 18 (1):72–83.

Elster, J. 2011. Procreative beneficence: cui bono? *Bioethics* 25 (9):482–8.

Goold, I., and J. Savulescu. 2009. In favour of freezing eggs for non-medical reasons. *Bioethics* 23 (1):47–58.

Harman, E. 2004. Can we harm and benefit in creating? *Philosophical Perspectives* 18:89–113.

Harris, John. 2001. One principle and three fallacies of disability studies. *Journal of Medical Ethics* 27 (6):383–7.

———. 2007. *Enhancing evolution: the ethical case for making better people*. Princeton, NJ: Princeton University Press.

———. 2009. Enhancements are a moral obligation. In *Human enhancement*, edited by J. Savulescu and N. Bostrom. New York: Oxford University Press.

Hauskeller, Michael. 2013. *Better humans? Understanding the enhancement project*. Durhan: Acumen.

Herissone-Kelly, P. 2006. Procreative beneficence and the prospective parent. *Journal of Medical Ethics* 32 (3):166–9.

Holm, S., and R. Bennett. 2014. The proper scope of the principle of procreative beneficence revisited. *Monash Bioethics Review* 32 (1–2):22–32.

Hotke, A. 2014. The principle of procreative beneficence: old arguments and a new challenge. *Bioethics* 28 (5):255–62.

Marcus, Ruth Barcan, 1980. Moral dilemmas and consistency. *The Journal of Philosophy*, 77: 121–136

Parfit, Derek. 1984. *Reasons and persons*. Oxford, UK: Clarendon Press.

Parker, M. 2007. The best possible child. *Journal of Medical Ethics* 33 (5):279–83.

Roberts, Melinda A., and David T. Wasserman. 2009. *Harming future persons: ethics, genetics and the nonidentity problem*. Vol. 35 of International Library of Ethics, Law, and the New Medicine. New York: Springer.

Savulescu, Julian. 2001a. In defense of selection for nondisease genes. *American Journal of Bioethics* 1 (1):16–9.

———. 2001b. Procreative beneficence: why we should select the best children. *Bioethics* 15 (5–6):413–26.

———. 2005. New breeds of humans: The moral obligation to enhance. *Reproductive Biomedicine Online* 10:36–39.

———. 2007. In defence of procreative beneficence. *Journal of Medical Ethics* 33 (5):284–8.

Savulescu, Julian, and Guy Kahane. 2009. The moral obligation to create children with the best chance of the best life. *Bioethics* 23 (5):274–90.

Sparrow, Robert. 2007. Procreative beneficence, obligation, and eugenics. *Genomics, Society and Policy* 3 (3):43–59.

———. 2011. A not-so-new eugenics: Harris and Savulescu on human enhancement. *Hastings Center Report* 41 (1):32–42.

———. 2012. Human enhancement and sexual dimorphism. *Bioethics* 26 (9):464–75.

Stoller, SE. 2008. Why we are not morally required to select the best children: a response to Savulescu. *Bioethics* 22 (7):364–9.

Strawson, Peter F. 1962. Freedom and resentment. *Proceedings of the British Academy* 48:1–25.

Urbanek, Valentina. 2013. The ethics of embryo selection. In *Designer biology: the ethics of intensively engineering biological and ecological systems*, edited by R. L. Sandler and J. Basl. Lanham, MD: Lexington Books.

Wilkinson, Richard G., and Kate Pickett. 2010. *The spirit level: why greater equality makes societies stronger*. New York: Bloomsbury Press.

Williams, Bernard. 1965. Ethical Consistency. *Proceedings of the Aristotelian Society* (Supplement), 39: 103–124.

Chapter 5

The Illusion of Control

Reprogenetic Technologies and the Natural Lottery

Introduction

One of the most common arguments in favor of reprogenetic technologies is their presumed ability to defy the lack of control implicit in the "natural lottery" that results from normal human reproduction. In fact, advocates of reprogenetics find sexual reproduction to be a rather imperfect mechanism for the creation of human beings. In a coauthored article, Savulescu and Harris declares sexual reproduction to be not only an inefficient activity but an unsafe one:

> Approximately 3–5% of babies born have some abnormality. Natural reproduction not only involves the foreseeable and unavoidable creation of some embryos that will die but also some embryos that will go on to become very disabled human beings. Many embryos created are so genetically abnormal that they die, but some survive only to die as grossly deformed babies. The branch of medicine known as "teratology" bears witness to the imperfection of natural reproduction—babies born with missing limbs, with

a missing brain, or with two heads (Savulescu and Harris 2004, 92).

Likewise, Harris (2015a) cites the following statistics from the March of Dimes:

> Every year an estimated 7.9 million children—6 percent of total births worldwide—are born with a serious birth defect of genetic or partially genetic origin. Additional hundreds of thousands more are born with serious birth defects of post-conception origin, including maternal exposure to environmental agents (teratogens) such as alcohol, rubella, syphilis and iodine deficiency that can harm a developing fetus (32).

He then declares sexual reproduction to be a "very dangerous activity indeed," one that

> involves genes being recklessly combined—sometimes literally but always figuratively—in the dark, with unforeseeable consequences for the resulting children, parents, and the generations to come (Harris 2015b, 5).

Reprogenetics advocates often contrast the dangers of sexual reproduction with the safe outcomes resulting from reprogenetic technologies (O'Donnell, 2014), and the vagaries of sexual reproduction with the rational control they believe is afforded by these technologies. For Savulescu, for instance:

> Our future is in our hands now, whether we like it or not. But by not allowing enhancement and control over the genetic nature of our offspring, we consign a person to the natural lottery, and now, by having the power to do otherwise, to fail to do otherwise is to be responsible for the results of the

natural lottery. We must make a choice: the natural lottery or rational choice (Savulescu 2005, 39).

Supporters of reprogenetics consider this presumed ability to control our offspring's characteristics a way to ensure that we improve on the not particularly impressive entities that human beings are. As Harris puts it:

In short, I propose both the wisdom and the necessity of intervening in what has been called the natural lottery of life, to improve things by taking control of evolution and our future development to the point, and indeed beyond the point, where we humans will have changed, perhaps into a new and certainly into a better species altogether (Harris 2007, 4).

Or, as Green confidently declares:

But what nature accomplished in the past by means of natural selection, we may do by direction. Emerging genetic technologies permit us to replace the destructive and wasteful process of natural selection with intelligence and design (Green 2007, 15).

Some critics of reprogenetic technologies have actually decried this determination to govern reproduction as a problematic desire to strive for mastery (President's Council on Bioethics 2003; Sandel 2007). For them, the attempt to control sexual reproduction constitutes a Promethean wish to remake human nature to serve our purposes and to satisfy our desires, or a hubristic attitude incapable of appreciating what is inherently good about humanity. In this chapter, I tackle the desire for mastery that is present in defenses of reprogenetic technologies.

I leave aside, however, the question of whether such striving is morally appropriate. My challenge to proponents' claims about the control that reprogenetic technologies will afford is two-fold. First, by proponents' own account, it is not at all clear that human beings have the intellectual wherewithal to aptly control the so-called natural lottery. If advocates of reprogenetics are to be believed, human wisdom is limited and thus it is doubtful that human beings should be trusted to suitably direct their own evolution. Second, even if one were to concede human beings' wisdom, I argue that the degree of control over the natural lottery that reprogenetic technologies are said to grant us is illusory, the result of misunderstanding human biology and the role of genetics.

Designing Human Beings: The Fool thinks he is Wise

In an article questioning Sandel's criticisms of reprogenetic technologies in general and enhancement techniques in particular, Frances Kamm (2005) called attention to what she believes is a serious concern.[1] She contended that what is worrying about reprogenetic technologies is not, pace Sandel, that they are motivated by people's desire to have control over their offspring or their unwillingness to accept what comes unbidden. Rather, what is troublesome about these technologies and the desire for control that they embody stems from human beings' lack of imagination as designers. She believes that, because most people's conception of what constitutes human goods is very limited, the results of human design will likely conform to a limited and predictable

---

1. Kamm also thinks that questions about safety and scarce resources constitute major problems with enhancement technologies.

set of goods. For her, in attempting to control reproduction and design our offspring, human beings are likely to restrict, rather than expand, the number and combination of goods that could exist if things were left to chance and thus to reduce the range of appreciation of human goods. As she instructively puts it:

> A parent who might have designed his child to have the good trait of composing classical music, could not have conceived that it would be good to have a child who turns out to be one of the Beatles. (To have conceived it, would have involved creating the style before the Beatles did.) (Kamm 2005, 14)

I want to call attention here to a related concern, one that stems directly from reprogenetics proponents' own assessment of human wisdom or lack thereof. Such an assessment arguably exposes a tension—or full-blown inconsistency—in some advocates' claims. On the one hand, reprogenetics advocates assert that we human beings would be better at designing our offspring than sexual reproduction and natural selection are. Indeed, they claim that reprogenetic technologies will allow prospective parents to control the mistakes of natural reproduction. As we have seen, they contend that such control will improve our lot, allowing us to live longer and healthier lives, boosting our intellectual capacities and talents, enhancing love and marriage, refining our emotional experiences, increasing our subjective sense of well-being, and ultimately building more productive societies. On the other hand, at least some reprogenetics supporters assert that our increasing ability to affect nature and ourselves might just produce the annihilation of our planet. They insist that unless we promote yet another type of enhancement—moral bioenhancement—the improvement of human beings' cognitive capacities (designed by us), together with current technological advances in the physical and the biological sciences (also designed by us), might just result in human demise (DeGrazia 2014; Persson and Savulescu 2008). As Persson and Savulescu ominously put it:

> The human species, and the rest of life on Earth, faces a series of disastrous threats. Some of these have been with us throughout our whole history. Scientific progress has helped us to protect ourselves against some of these, and will probably help us to protect ourselves against more in the future. But the irony is that the very same progress creates other equally lethal threats. . . .[I]n order to reduce the existential threat that cognitive enhancement poses, we require a moral enhancement, an enhancement of our motivation to act morally. The threats come not only from cognitive enhancement by novel biomedical and genetic means, but also from the growth of knowledge by traditional cultural means, and by external means, such as access to supercomputers. Indeed, it may be that we already are too cognitively advanced for our own good (and for the good of other species on Earth) (167).

Likewise, DeGrazia (2014) describes our sorry state of affairs as follows:

> The status quo is deeply problematic because there is such an abundance of immoral behaviour, with devastating consequences, and serious risk of worse to come. Consider examples. In the 1990s, genocides occurred in Rwanda and Bosnia. . . . Slavery still exists. . . . Forced prostitution and participation in pornography, often involving children, is a reality. . . . Around the world, violence and other forms of oppression are committed against girls and women, religious and ethnic minorities, and others who are considered

'outside' the group committing the violence.... An estimated 850 million people are chronically undernourished, ... 2.6 billion lack access to basic sanitation, ... 2 billion lack electricity.... In response to such pervasive severe poverty—and despite being causally implicated in much of it—leaders of developed countries fail to provide the modest levels of foreign assistance that could contribute greatly towards solving these problems.... At the same time, the USA commits far greater sums to subsidies and tax breaks for those who don't need them. Nor, with few exceptions, do individuals contribute substantially to prevent these preventable deaths and subhuman living conditions (362).

Now, the claim that creatures foolish enough to put their own existence at risk should be trusted taking control of human reproduction and designing future human beings certainly requires justification. If human injudiciousness has led us to develop technologies capable of annihilating the human species and destroying the planet and our inherent immorality has led us to commit all sorts of atrocities, why would one believe that those same humans would be wise enough to direct human evolution in appropriate ways? At the least, claims that our rational choices are surely better than the natural lottery in designing our offspring require defense. After all, we are responsible for the technologies we have developed and implemented and for the ways in which we use them, and we are also responsible for the policies that have given rise to the current status quo that is decried (appropriately so) by reprogenetic proponents and used to justify the need for moral bioenhancements. True, one could object that the "natural lottery" has created us—with our injudiciousness— and that trying to control this process might therefore result in wiser creatures. Nonetheless, insofar as our wisdom is in question, there is no obvious reason to believe that we would do a better job than the natural lottery in creating wiser beings.

Misunderstanding Human Biology: Plant a Radish, Get a Radish

Debates about reprogenetic technologies present these technologies as smoothly and surely evolving from determining the presence or absence of a particular genetic mutation or variant or tinkering with an embryo's genome to having a child with or without a particular phenotypic trait. Concerns about human beings' lack of imagination or wisdom accept this picture-perfect view and grant that reprogenetic technologies will allow human beings to control—even if they do so poorly—the genetic nature of our offspring and ultimately the direction of human evolution. In this section, I contest this assumption. I argue that, even if human beings were wise and imaginative enough to appropriately direct the creation of future people, it is unlikely that the use of reprogenetic technologies will permit us to wrest control over sexual reproduction. This is so for at least two reasons: First, the mechanisms of sexual reproduction do not stop operating when reprogenetic technologies are used, and second, multiple factors—and not just genetic ones—play a role in the creation of a human being as well as in the direction of evolution.

Reprogenetic Technologies: The "Dangers" of Sexual Reproduction without the (Fun of) Sex

As we saw earlier, reprogenetics advocates believe sexual reproduction to be a perilous activity, one that results not only in embryo destruction and the birth of individuals with a variety of genetically influenced diseases and disabilities but ultimately in the creation of very imperfect beings. Their claim is that rational interventions in the so-called natural lottery, facilitated by the use of reprogenetic technologies, will be able to reduce or fully eliminate the various hazards that result from sexual reproduction.

Of course, this is simply nonsense—at least regarding the reprogenetic technologies currently in use. First, sexual reproduction mechanisms, the "reckless" combination of genes that proponents decry, take place whether or not reprogenetic technologies are utilized. Meiotic recombination, which leads to the formation of gametes with various novel combinations of the parental genotypes, occur during the formation of the parental egg and sperm. Fertilization then leads to pairing of the gametes' recombinant genomes. These processes are unaffected by the reprogenetic technologies currently in use. As described in chapter 2, in vitro fertilization (IVF) involves the retrieval of post-recombination gametes and thus presents all the "dangers" of sexual reproduction without the sex. Preimplantation genetic diagnosis (PGD), on the other hand, is a diagnostic or screening technology usually involving embryos (i.e., after meiotic recombination and fertilization have occurred). Even when it is used to evaluate gametes, it, also, has no effect on recombination processes. Certainly, PGD can result in the selection of particular embryos because they have or lack certain characteristics, and perhaps it could, at least in theory, allow for the intentional selection of specific combinations of traits, but it has no influence on genetic recombination per se. Evidence that current reprogenetic technologies do not have much influence on the "unsafe" process of sexual reproduction includes the fact that the percentage of children born with congenital malformations is not reduced, compared with unassisted pregnancies, when these technologies are used (Parazzini et al. 2015). In fact, an increasing amount of evidence suggests that children conceived through these technologies are at a higher risk of birth defects than children born naturally (Hansen et al. 2013; Heisey et al. 2015; Qin et al. 2015).

It is true that the use of PGD can help prevent the birth of individuals with a variety of genetically influenced conditions, but this is a far cry from achieving control over sexual reproduction. Tests for many congenital malformations do not exist, and there is no evidence that they are likely to exist for all such conditions. Moreover, if, as some research indicates, reprogenetic technologies contribute to a higher risk of malformation, it would be puzzling to suggest the use of PGD—which requires IVF and other related techniques—as a way to avoid the health risks produced, at least in part, by such technologies. Furthermore, although some studies have suggested that PGD does not increase congenital anomalies or other health problems (Banerjee et al. 2008; Liebaers et al. 2010), more and larger studies are needed to corroborate such results.

Likewise, if gene editing techniques could one day be used to address particular genetic mutations implicated in diseases and disabilities, they would have little effect on recombination processes related to sexual reproduction. These technologies are applied before conception (i.e., to gametes) and perhaps could correct at least some undesired recombinations, but they could not control error processes that occur during fertilization. Alternatively, if they were applied after the embryos are created, they could solve only genetic problems that could be diagnosed at that stage. Theoretically, gene editing could be used at both stages, but given the other problems discussed later, it is hard to see that attempts to control the natural lottery could justify this use of resources. Whether or not the use of gene editing technologies will give rise to birth defects and other health problems in humans is, at this point, unknown. But given the complexity of human biology, such a possibility does not seem implausible.

Human cloning—were it ever proven to be an effective and safe reproductive technique—would indeed affect sexual reproduction mechanisms because it would allow fertilization after the transfer of an adult cell nucleus to an unfertilized egg. But reproductive cloning is unlikely to become the reproductive technology of choice for most people. More importantly, it is not clear that cloning is a particularly rational way to guide evolution because it limits diversity of the gene pool and thus decreases the chances that future human beings could adapt to novel environments. After all, as much as proponents decry "the destructive and wasteful process of natural selection," it will not stop working simply because some dislike its results. Cloning might theoretically produce individuals with carefully selected genomes, but natural selection will still act on those genomes (i.e., by means of differential reproductive success) in response to environmental pressures.

Equally nonsensical is proponents' suggestion that reprogenetic technologies would have any influence on birth defects of postconception origin, such as those resulting from maternal exposure to alcohol, iodine deficiency, or certain pathogens (e.g., rubella, syphilis) that can harm a developing fetus. Of course, many of these birth defects might come to be treated or cured at some point as a result of biomedical developments, but that will have slight effect on sexual recombination mechanisms.

Given this situation, advocates' enthusiasm for the ability of reprogenetic technologies to eliminate the "dangers" of sexual reproduction and intervene in the natural lottery to control human evolution seems misplaced. Let me reiterate that this does not mean that reprogenetic technologies cannot be used to reduce some genetically influenced diseases and disabilities and perhaps at some point to create children with particular phenotypic traits unrelated to disease, but this is likely to have little effect on the multiple and varied quirks of sexual reproduction—and in regard to cloning, it is unlikely to constitute an advantage over sexual reproduction. So much, then, for controlling the hazards of sexual reproduction and natural selection through the use of reprogenetics.

When You Are a Hammer, Everything Looks like a Nail

A second reason to doubt proponents' claims regarding our ability to control the natural lottery of sexual reproduction and natural selection through reprogenetics is that beliefs about such control are the result of scientific misunderstandings. Recall that PGD and gene editing techniques attend exclusively to molecular components. PGD offers information about the presence or absence of certain genetic mutations or variants, whereas gene editing techniques allow DNA to be inserted, replaced, or removed from a genome. Decisions about what children to bring or not bring into the world, however, are grounded on the assumption that they will or will not have particular *phenotypic* traits. Reprogenetics proponents' concerns about the dangers of sexual reproduction stem from the fact that it results in phenotypic traits that they believe may decrease people's well-being. Similarly, their desire to control reproductive processes arises out of a wish to create children with phenotypic traits that proponents consider likely to make the lives of those children—and perhaps of others—better.

But these ambitions of control are grounded on an untenable genetic determinism. To be sure, reprogenetics advocates do not explicitly embrace genetic determinism. On the contrary, they are eager to reject such doctrine (Green 2007, 81–9; Harris 2007, 127; Savulescu et al. 2006; Silver 1997, 367). For instance, in an article defending selection against criminal dispositions, Savulescu and colleagues plainly states:

> Both parents who overestimate their child's likely actions, and law enforcement agencies who underestimate a person's likely behaviour based on their genes, would be acting on a deterministic understanding of genetics which is false. Even if a deterministic account of behaviour is true, genetics forms only one cause from a very long list of causes which lead to any given behaviour. Our genes, therefore, do not determine our behaviour, even when they are in fact producing known behaviour-altering chemical effect (Savulescu et al. 2006, 166).

In spite of proponents' explicit repudiation of genetic determinism, though, it is difficult to see how their control motivations could make any sense without such an assumption. One might charitably agree that proponents' ambition to control does not necessitate some versions of genetic determinism, such as the "complete information" kind, which affirms that our genes dictate everything about us, or the "intervention is useless" type, which asserts that for traits that have a genetic component, intervention is powerless (Kaplan 2000, 11–2). But some form of determinism must be at play in proponents' dreams of controlling sexual reproduction, and ultimately human evolution, by means of reprogenetic technologies. The degree of influence to which proponents aspire appears possible with these technologies only if one assumes that selection and enhancement practices will reliably have the desired outcomes. If highly predictable results cannot be reasonably guaranteed, then it is hard to see how one might be able to exercise such a degree of control over the dangerous activity that sexual reproduction is said to be.

The focus on genetic aspects found in reprogenetics defenses is, of course, consistent with societal values that emphasize efficiency, control, and quick fixes. Genomic factors provide us with some explanatory and predictive power for a variety of human traits. And thanks to our technologies, some of these genetic factors can be identified, silenced, knocked-out, edited, spliced, and otherwise manipulated, allowing us a certain level of command, particularly in laboratories. Thus, in contrast to extragenomic elements (e.g., social, environmental), genomic factors appear relatively easy to manage. Of course, the fact that we have focused our resources on trying to understand genomic factors has something to do with our beliefs both in the salience of genetic factors and in the tractability of those factors and the intractability of environmental and social ones (de Melo-Martin 2005).

Proponents of reprogenetics' wishful thinking notwithstanding, the path from genotype to phenotype is anything but straightforward. This in no way means, of course, that people's genetic endowment has nothing to do with the traits usually discussed by reprogenetics proponents, such as certain diseases and disabilities, character and cognitive traits, and physical characteristics. Neither does it mean that it is impossible to say something meaningful and appropriate about the causal roles of genes in the development of phenotypic traits. However, reprogenetic technologies make genetic aspects salient at the exclusion of all other factors. It might well be the case that such salience is appropriate for some human traits, but it is beyond dispute that for most human diseases, and indeed for the majority of the traits that populate defenses of reprogenetic technologies (e.g., aggression, alcoholism, antisocial personality, memory and intelligence, novelty seeking, substance addiction), the emphasis given to genetics is completely mistaken.

Current scientific knowledge clearly contradicts any deterministic understanding of human biology. The biomedical sciences are providing us with information that disputes any claims about reducing human phenotypic traits to the influence of simple—or even not so simple—genetic markers. Contributions of genetic factors to complex traits are neither necessary nor sufficient to produce the traits in question. This is also true for complex diseases and disorders that represent the greatest health burdens, such as cardiovascular disease, type 2 diabetes, autoimmune diseases, cancer, and neurological diseases. Indeed, because of the phenomenon of reduced penetrance, whereby individuals with a particular disease-causing mutation fail to express most or all features of the disease in question, it is also the case even for many monogenic diseases (Cooper et al. 2013). Reduced or incomplete penetrance can be a function of the specific mutations involved or of allele dosage. It may also stem from differential allelic expression, which may be influenced by age or sex, and it can reflect the actions of unlinked modifier genes, epigenetic changes, and environmental factors.

Multiple genes at different loci contribute to complex diseases and other traits, and those loci may be interacting with each other. Because of the common phenomenon of pleiotropy, a single causal mutation or variant may be related to multiple phenotypes, or multiple variants in the same gene or locus may be associated with different phenotypes (Solovieff et al. 2013). Depending on their roles in the pathogenesis of diseases, interactions among various alleles or loci may be additive, multiplicative, or without additional effect. Modifier genetic elements can also interact with mutations involved in the production of some diseases. Despite our increasing technological power to find genetic factors that influence complex diseases and traits, the results actually evince the staggering complexity of human biology (Barr and Misener 2016; Eichler et al. 2010; Ritchie 2015; Witte, Visscher, and Wray 2014; Zhu et al. 2015).

Moreover, epigenetic processes such as DNA methylation, histone modifications, and RNA interference can change the expression patterns of genes without altering the DNA sequence (Barr and Misener 2016; Eissenberg 2014; Martos, Tang, and Wang 2015). Epigenetic modifications contribute to the differential regulation of gene expression, to imprinting—which results in differences in gene expression depending on the allele's parental origin, and to gene silencing, all of which can impact the path from genotype to phenotype. More and more evidence shows that the epigenome, the combination of changes affecting gene expression in a cell, is of astounding complexity. Furthermore, epigenetic modifications can be passed, on not only from cell to cell as cells divide, but in certain cases also from one generation to the next (Martos, Tang, and Wang 2015). To make matters more complicated, lifestyle and environmental factors (e.g., smoking, stress, malnutrition, exposure to harmful chemicals) can subject individuals to pressures that induce epigenetic changes which might result in a variety of diseases and affect behavioral traits. Evidence shows that epigenomic changes are involved in neurodevelopmental disorders and intellectual disabilities; they have been linked to physical and developmental abnormalities; and they can result in neurodegenerative diseases, immunodeficiency, congenital heart disease, autism spectrum disorders, and cancer (Hoffmann, Zimmermann, and Spengler 2015; Mirabella, Foster, and Bartke 2015). Additionally, the expression of most human diseases involves complex causal interactions among genomic, organismic, and environmental factors (Chung et al. 2013; Jackson 2014; Lee, Kim, and Park 2015; Pasipoularides 2015).

Of course, at least some diseases or disorders involve not just biological facts but also are influenced by the particular social and environmental context in which those traits are expressed. Consider, for instance, dyslexia (a difficulty in learning to read), a disorder that some reprogenetic advocates argue may come to be understood as a genetic problem that can be routinely screened for and selected against or genetically modified (Green 2007, 79). Evidence shows that this disorder, which, particularly when identified early, can be successfully corrected or even prevented, has some apparently complex genetic component (Mascheretti et al. 2015). Nonetheless, the presence of associated genetic (or neurological) markers can result in a very different phenotypic expression depending on the language spoken. For some speakers of languages such as Italian, Spanish, Chinese, or Japanese who have neurological deficits consistent with dyslexia, reading accuracy constitutes only a minor problem. However, the problem can be a significant one for speakers of other languages such as English or French (Paulesu et al. 2001). The importance of the social and institutional context is even more obvious in regard to many disabilities. As many have argued, the effect that disability can have on a person's well-being is dependent not only on the disability in question but particularly on the social context in which such disability is experienced (Asch 1999, 2003; Barnes 2014; Goering 2008; Parens and Asch 1999; Scully 2008; Shakespeare 2006; Wasserman and Asch 2006). Although these considerations do not impugn proponents' aspirations of control (after all, one could indeed select or enhance dyslexia genetic factors or whatever mutations or epigenetic modifications might be involved in some disabilities), they do undermine the grounds for such control. If many diseases and disabilities do not necessarily lower well-being, then the rationale for attempting to avoid the "dangers" of sexual reproduction seems less obvious.

If the dream of control is untenable when considering most diseases and disorders that affect human beings, it is even more so regarding the overwhelming majority, if not all, of the traits that are the staple of reprogenetics defenses. As we have seen, such traits include intelligence, gender, empathy, sense of humor, optimism, novelty seeking, shyness, physical beauty, self-control, and moral character, among others. To begin with, these traits involve entities that are difficult to specify meaningfully in a quantitative manner. Therefore, it is unclear how a genotype can be selected or manipulated in order to obtain these particular phenotypes. A variety of value judgments play an essential, ine-liminable role in the characterization of these traits. Of course, some genetic factors can contribute to what are usually under-stood as instances of these traits in an individual, but that is far from providing us with a reliable manner of obtaining these phe-notypes by simply selecting certain genetic markers or manipu-lating the genome.

This problem affects even traits that are thought to be well characterized. For instance, I have already mentioned in chapter 3 the concerns raised by using reprogenetic technolo-gies for "gender" selection. As we saw there, what these tech-nologies can accomplish is the identification of chromosomal sex. Chromosomal sex, however, is not even determinative of anatomical or physiological sex (Öçal 2011), much less of the attitudes, behaviors, and roles often associated with a particular gender (Butler 2004; Caplan and Caplan 2009; Fausto-Sterling 1992, 2000). But a child of a particular gender is precisely what parents choosing sex selection ultimately want and what repro-genetic technologies are supposed to deliver: a way to defy the natural lottery. Nonetheless, whatever the relationships between biological sex and the normative psychological and behavioral characteristics associated with a particular gender, it is clear that biology is not determinative of gender characteristics.

Similar issues arise with other phenotypic traits that pro-ponents claim reprogenetic technologies can select or enhance. Take, for instance, aggression. To claim that PGD can or will be able to identify genetic mutations or variants involved in aggression is to presuppose that determinations of such a trait are independent of the way in which it is characterized and judged. But this is absurd. In a particular social setting, the same behavior can be judged as either appropriately forceful or aggressive. Consider, for example, the different characteriza-tions of an energetic exchange when the participants are a man and a woman, or a white man and an African-American man. Moreover, although advocates of reprogenetics use the concepts of aggression and criminal or antisocial behavior interchangeably (Savulescu et al. 2006), such identification again ignores the roles of normative judgments and social context in characterizing these very complex traits. Criminal or antisocial behaviors are social categories, not genetic ones, so it is not completely clear what it means to say that there are associations between some genetic mutations and criminal tendencies (Savulescu et al. 2006). It might well be that all known societies have characterized certain behaviors as criminal or antisocial (e.g., killing human beings under certain conditions). But even in those cases, complex value judgments are at stake. In many other instances, behaviors that are characterized as criminal in one culture would not be so understood in another or at a different time in human history; examples include the use of recreational drugs, prostitution, blasphemy, and engaging in homosexual acts. Analogous arguments can be offered in relation to the other many traits that are presented by proponents of reprogenetics as amenable to genetic selection or enhancement and as very much under people's control.

Why it Matters

Showing that the control advocated by proponents is unattainable is important for multiple reasons. First, and most obvious, is the fact that the deterministic view that grounds their ambitions of control fails to offer an adequate description of the complexity of human traits. If having an adequate understanding of human biology is important for public participation and policy formation, then such an incorrect view contributes to uninformed public discussions and can lead to problematic public policies.

Second, the touted possibility of control can contribute to a misunderstanding of what prospective parents can achieve through reprogenetic technologies. It is true, for at least some traits, that insofar as prospective parents select against the trait, they eliminate the possibility that their offspring will have it. Think, for instance, of prospective parents' use of PGD to identify embryos with the mutation for Huntington's disease so as to select those embryos that lack the mutation. As I have said, however, the majority of the traits that are considered as possible candidates for selection or enhancement are not like the Huntington's disease trait, which is caused by a single gene and is thought to have almost complete penetrance (i.e., anyone who has this particular genetic mutation, and who lives long enough, will develop the disease) (ACMG/ASHG 1998).[2] Nonetheless, the emphasis on the control that reprogenetic technologies presumably will afford us might lead prospective parents to believe that other traits are equally manageable. That, however, would be mistaken.

Third, presenting human traits as if they were exclusively the result of the play of our genetic endowment and completely independent of our social life and value judgments limits the range of solutions that can be offered to the problems that reprogenetic technologies presumably aim to address. We would do well to remember that the ultimate goal these technologies ostensibly will help us achieve is the improvement of human well-being. Even if genetic factors are important contributors to human phenotypic traits and reprogenetic technologies can be useful to select and enhance some of those traits, such factors are not the

2. Noticeably, however, the penetrance of Huntington's disease depends on the number of CAG repeats in the huntingtin gene. Although for expansions of greater than 39 repeats the Huntington phenotype seems to have complete penetrance, individuals with a repeat length of 27 to 35 might have a normal phenotype. Moreover, the severity of the disease and the age at onset seem to be affected by a variety of factors (Panegyres et al. 2015).

only important ones. If, for instance, the social context in which human traits are expressed is relevant to their characterization, then changes to our social, political, and legal systems can also accomplish at least some of the aims that reprogenetic technologies seek to obtain.

For example, the desire to select for or to enhance particular traits often results from the fact that such traits confer a competitive advantage in our society. Take, for instance, the desire to enhance human height or to choose the sex of a child (the latter now being technologically possible). There is little doubt that the value of these traits depends on our particular social arrangements and not on the fact that being tall or having a particular sex necessarily increases one's well-being regardless of the kind of society humans create. Indeed, our social arrangements do result in unjustifiable disadvantages for people who are short or are female and in undeserved rewards for people who are tall or are males. It is in this context that we may believe selection or enhancement of these traits would increase our children's well-being, leading at least some to attempt to control the vagaries of sexual reproduction. Attending to the social context, however, would give us another way of addressing such desires, one that arguably has other advantages too. Changing our social arrangements and institutions so as to ensure that gender or height, for instance, does not constitute a source of unjustifiable benefits or hindrances will also contribute to increasing the well-being of children whose parents cannot use, or choose not to use, reprogenetic technologies.

Conclusion

Advocates of reprogenetic technologies deride sexual reproduction and natural evolution as wasteful and dangerous. They believe that reprogenetic technologies provide a more rational and appropriate way to create human beings and direct their evolution. In this chapter, I have shown that such ambitions of control are undesirable and illusory. Human beings' lack of imagination about basic goods, and particularly the lack of wisdom recognized by proponents themselves, calls into question the advisability of trying to control the natural lottery to the degree proponents wish. Furthermore, even if such an amount of control were desirable, it would be unachievable through these technologies. Most reprogenetic technologies, and certainly those now in widespread use, do not affect sexual reproduction or evolutionary processes and thus cannot preclude a variety of congenital problems that proponents claim can be managed. Furthermore, an untenable genetic determinism underlies proponents' beliefs about the control that reprogenetic technologies can provide.

To be sure, the genetic revolution has made genetic or genomic aspects salient and in so doing has resulted in a variety of epistemic and practical successes.[3] But this does not mean that genomic factors are all that matters, much less that tinkering with these factors will reliably produce the kinds of outcomes some might wish. This is not to say that reprogenetic technologies afford us no control whatsoever over human phenotypic traits. They certainly give prospective parents a significant amount of influence over the children they are willing to bring into the world, but such control can hardly be said to eliminate the so-called burdens of sexual reproduction. Of course, the fact that the control reprogenetic technologies can give prospective parents will be limited might have little effect on their use. After all, people often utilize their time and money for all

---

3. Such successes are, unsurprisingly, often used as a reason for rejecting concerns about the excessive attention given to genomics when trying to understand a variety of aspects related to human well-being.

sorts of activities that prove useless or of limited effectiveness. Surely, though, proponents' exaggerated claims about the power of reprogenetic technologies are unlikely to make matters better.

References

(ACMG/ASHG) American College of Medical Genetics/American Society of Human Genetics Huntington Disease Genetic Testing Working Group. 1998. ACMG/ASHG statement: laboratory guidelines for Huntington disease genetic testing. *American Journal of Human Genetics* 62 (5):1243–7.

Asch, Adrienne. 1999. Prenatal diagnosis and selective abortion: a challenge to practice and policy. *American Journal of Public Health* 89 (11):1649–57.

———. 2003. Disability equality and prenatal testing: contradictory or compatible? *Florida State University Law Review* 30 (2):315–42.

Banerjee, I., M. Shevlin, M. Taranissi, A. Thornhill, H. Abdalla, O. Ozturk, J. Barnes, and A. Sutcliffe. 2008. Health of children conceived after preimplantation genetic diagnosis: a preliminary outcome study. *Reproductive Biomedicine Online* 16 (3):376–81.

Barnes, Elizabeth. 2014. Valuing disability, causing disability. *Ethics* 125 (1):88–113.

Barr, C. L., and V. L. Misener. 2016. Decoding the non-coding genome: elucidating genetic risk outside the coding genome. *Genes Brain Behavior* 15(1):187–204.

Butler, Judith. 2004. *Undoing gender.* New York: Routledge.

Caplan, Paula J., and Jeremy B. Caplan. 2009. *Thinking critically about research on sex and gender.* 3rd ed. Boston: Pearson/Allyn and Bacon.

Chung, S. J., S. M. Armasu, K. J. Anderson, J. M. Biernacka, T. G. Lesnick, D. N. Rider, J. M. Cunningham, J. E. Ahlskog, R. Frigerio, and D. M. Maraganore. 2013. Genetic susceptibility loci, environmental exposures, and Parkinson's disease: a case-control study of gene-environment interactions. *Parkinsonism and Related Disorders* 19 (6):595–9.

Cooper, D. N., M. Krawczak, C. Polychronakos, C. Tyler-Smith, and H. Kehrer-Sawatzki. 2013. Where genotype is not predictive of phenotype: towards an understanding of the molecular basis of reduced penetrance in human inherited disease. *Human Genetics* 132 (10):1077–130.

DeGrazia, David. 2014. Moral enhancement, freedom, and what we (should) value in moral behaviour. *Journal of Medical Ethics* 40 (6):361–68.

de Melo-Martin, Inmaculada. 2005. *Taking biology seriously: what biology can and cannot tell us about moral and public policy issues.* Lanham, MD: Rowman & Littlefield.

Eichler, E. E., J. Flint, G. Gibson, A. Kong, S. M. Leal, J. H. Moore, and J. H. Nadeau. 2010. Missing heritability and strategies for finding the underlying causes of complex disease. *Nature Review Genetics* 11 (6):446–50.

Eissenberg, J.C. 2014. Epigenetics: modifying the genetic blueprint. Missouri medicine 111 (5):428–33.

Fausto-Sterling, Anne. 1992. *Myths of gender: biological theories about women and men.* 2nd ed. New York: BasicBooks.

———. 2000. *Sexing the body: gender politics and the construction of sexuality.* 1st ed. New York: Basic Books.

Goering, Sara. 2008. 'You say you're happy, but...': contested quality of life judgments in bioethics and disability studies. *Journal of Bioethical Inquiry* 5 (2–3):125–35.

Green, Ronald Michael. 2007. *Babies by design: the ethics of genetic choice.* New Haven, CT: Yale University Press.

Hansen, Michele, Jennifer J. Kurinczuk, Elizabeth Milne, Nicholas de Klerk, and Carol Bower. 2013. Assisted reproductive technology and birth defects: a systematic review and meta-analysis. *Human Reproduction Update* 19 (4):330–53.

Harris, John. 2007. *Enhancing evolution: the ethical case for making better people.* Princeton, NJ: Princeton University Press.

———. 2015a. Germline manipulation and our future worlds. *American Journal of Bioethics* 15 (12):30–4.

———. 2015b. Germline modification and the burden of human existence. *Cambridge Quarterly of Healthcare Ethics* 25 (1):6–18.

Heisey, Angela S., Erin M. Bell, Michele L. Herdt-Losavio, and Charlotte Druschel. 2015. Surveillance of congenital malformations in infants conceived through assisted reproductive technology or other fertility treatments. *Birth Defects Research Part A: Clinical and Molecular Teratology* 103 (2):119–26.

Hoffmann, A., C. A. Zimmermann, and D. Spengler. 2015. Molecular epigenetic switches in neurodevelopment in health and disease. *Frontiers in Behavioral Neuroscience* 9:120.

Jackson, F. L. 2014. Gene-environment interactions in human health: case studies and strategies for developing new paradigms and research methodologies. *Frontiers in Genetics* 5:271.

Kamm, Frances M. 2005. Is there a problem with enhancement? *American Journal of Bioethics* 5 (3):5–14.

Kaplan, Jonathan Michael. 2000. *The limits and lies of human genetic research: dangers for social policy*. New York: Routledge.

Lee, J. U., J. D. Kim, and C. S. Park. 2015. Gene-environment interactions in asthma: genetic and epigenetic effects. *Yonsei Medical Journal* 56 (4):877–86.

Liebaers, I., S. Desmyttere, W. Verpoest, M. De Rycke, C. Staessen, K. Sermon, P. Devroey, P. Haentjens, and M. Bonduelle. 2010. Report on a consecutive series of 581 children born after blastomere biopsy for preimplantation genetic diagnosis. *Human Reproduction* 25 (1):275–82.

Martos, S. N., W. Y. Tang, and Z. Wang. 2015. Elusive inheritance: transgenerational effects and epigenetic inheritance in human environmental disease. *Progress in Biophysics and Molecular Biology* 118 (1–2):44–54.

Mascheretti, S., A. Bureau, V. Trezzi, R. Giorda, and C. Marino. 2015. An assessment of gene-by-gene interactions as a tool to unfold missing heritability in dyslexia. *Human Genetics* 134 (7):749–60.

Mirabella, A. C., B. M. Foster, and T. Bartke. 2015. Chromatin deregulation in disease. *Chromosoma* 125 (1):75–93.

Öçal, G. 2011. Current concepts in disorders of sexual development. *Journal of Clinical Research in Pediatric Endocrinology* 3 (3):105–14.

O'Donnell, Norah. 2014. Breeding out disease. *60 Minutes*, CBS, October 26.

Panegyres, P. K., C. C. Shu, H. Y. Chen, and J. S. Paulsen. 2015. Factors influencing the clinical expression of intermediate CAG repeat length mutations of the Huntington's disease gene. *Journal of Neurology* 262 (2):277–84.

Parazzini, F., S. Cipriani, G. Bulfoni, C. Bulfoni, A. Frigerio, E. Somigliana, and F. Mosca. 2015. The risk of birth defects after assisted reproduction. *Journal of Assisted Reproductive Genetics* 32 (3):379–85.

Parens, Eirk, and Adrienne Asch. 1999. The disability rights critique of prenatal genetic testing: reflections and recommendations. *The Hastings Center Report* 29 (5):S1–22.

Pasipoularides, A. 2015. Linking genes to cardiovascular diseases: gene action and gene-environment interactions. *Journal of Cardiovascular Translational Research* 8 (9):506–27.

Paulesu, E., J. F. Démonet, F. Fazio, et al. 2001. Dyslexia: cultural diversity and biological unity. *Science* 291 (5511):2165–7.

Persson, I., and J. Savulescu. 2008. The perils of cognitive enhancement and the urgent imperative to enhance the moral character of humanity. *Journal of Applied Philosophy* 25 (3):162–7.

President's Council on Bioethics. 2003. *Beyond therapy: biotechnology and the pursuit of happiness.* 1st ed. New York: ReganBooks.

Qin, J., X. Sheng, H. Wang, D. Liang, H. Tan, and J. Xia. 2015. Assisted reproductive technology and risk of congenital malformations: a meta-analysis based on cohort studies. *Archives of Gynecology and Obstetrics* 292 (4):777–98.

Ritchie, M. D. 2015. Finding the epistasis needles in the genome-wide haystack. *Methods Molecular Biology* 1253:19–33.

Sandel, Michael J. 2007. *The case against perfection: ethics in the age of genetic engineering.* Cambridge, MA: Belknap Press of Harvard University Press.

Savulescu, Julian. 2005. New breeds of humans: the moral obligation to enhance. *Reproductive Biomedicine Online* 10:36–9.

Savulescu, Julian, and John Harris. 2004. The creation lottery: final lessons from natural reproduction—why those who accept natural reproduction should accept cloning and other Frankenstein reproductive technologies. *Cambridge Quarterly of Healthcare Ethics* 13 (1):90–5.

Savulescu, J., M. Hemsley, A. Newson, and B. Foddy. 2006. Behavioural genetics: why eugenic selection is preferable to enhancement. *Journal of Applied Philosophy* 23 (2):157–71.

Scully, Jackie Leach. 2008. *Disability bioethics: moral bodies, moral difference.* Feminist Constructions. Lanham, MD: Rowman & Littlefield.

Shakespeare, Tom. 2006. *Disability rights and wrongs.* New York: Routledge.

Silver, Lee M. 1997. *Remaking Eden: cloning and beyond in a brave new world*. 1st ed. New York: Avon Books.

Solovieff, N., C. Cotsapas, P. H. Lee, S. M. Purcell, and J. W. Smoller. 2013. Pleiotropy in complex traits: challenges and strategies. *Nature Review Genetics* 14 (7):483–95.

Wasserman, David, and Adrienne Asch. 2006. The uncertain rationale for prenatal disability screening. *The Virtual Mentor: VM* 8 (1):53–6.

Witte, J. S., P. M. Visscher, and N. R. Wray. 2014. The contribution of genetic variants to disease depends on the ruler. *Nature Review Genetics* 15 (11):765–76.

Zhu, Z., A. Bakshi, A. A. Vinkhuyzen, et al. 2015. Dominance genetic variation contributes little to the missing heritability for human complex traits. *American Journal of Human Genetics* 96 (3):377–85.

Chapter 6

Not of Woman Born

Reprogenetics and the Erasing of Women

Introduction

Approximately 1.6 million cycles of in vitro fertilization (IVF)
(ESHRE 2014), and 100,000 oocyte donation cycles (Weissman
et al. 2014) are performed annually worldwide. Millions of children have been born with the help of these technologies. Women's
bodies and women's reproductive materials are essential for the
development and implementation of reprogenetic technologies.
Women provide the eggs needed. They receive the hormonal
injections, undergo the surgeries, and suffer the physical and
psychological side effects associated with the use of these procedures. They gestate, give birth to, and usually rear the babies
who have been conceived, and in some cases selected, with the
help of such technologies. And if enhancement is ever going to
take place, it will be possible only with the critical participation
of women. Women bear a disproportionate share of the risks and
burdens involved in the use of reprogrenetics. And it is often said
that it is in the name of expanding women's reproductive choices
that these technologies are being developed.

Nonetheless, when reading prominent defenses of reprogenetic technologies, one might be forgiven for failing to notice

the essential role that women play. It is not only that feminist insights—along with feminist literature in the area—are conspicuously missing in mainstream defenses of reprogenetic technologies. It is also that influential proponents such as Harris, Savulescu, and Silver scarcely mention women in any substantive way when defending these technologies, and they appear completely oblivious to the burdens that these technologies impose on women's health and lives. Indeed, an analysis that takes gender seriously is strikingly absent in the works of the most prominent authors advocating for the use of these technologies—all of whom, perhaps not accidentally, are men.

In this chapter, I call attention to this absence and show its problematic consequences both for women and for any ethically sound analysis of reprogenetics. I begin by giving a brief overview of the gender-neutral analysis that proponents of reprogenetics employ. I then show the various ways in which the neglect of the gendered nature of reprogenetic decisions has negative impacts on women.

On Couples and Single Reproducers

It is not uncommon when discussing reprogenetic advances to talk about infertile couples, parents' rights and responsibilities, or gamete donors. The principle of procreative beneficence (PB), a principle (as we have seen in chapter 4) that entails a moral obligation to use reprogenetic technologies, explicitly refers to "couples" and "single reproducers" and fails to mention women at all. In fact, the 2001 and 2009 articles by Savulescu and colleagues in which PB is defended refer to women a total of 11 times, half of them involving discussions of cases in which women are presented as having to make reproductive decisions (which the authors take to be intuitively obvious) about whether to have a healthy or a sick child. In the other instances in which women are mentioned, it is either to argue that the possibility of increasing discrimination against women is not a sufficient reason against selecting the best child (Savulescu 2001, 424) or to indicate that PB instructs women to seriously consider IVF even when the expected well-being of the future child would be only negligibly better than if natural conception were used (Savulescu and Kahane 2009, 281). If one were expecting to find a discussion of the implications of instructing women to proceed in this way, one would be sorely disappointed. A typical example of the erasure of women in these authors' works is the following description of prenatal genetic testing:

> The most accessible reliable prenatal method is chorionic villous sampling (CVS) at about 11 weeks gestation, which provides both anatomical information about the fetus and genetic information. At 11 weeks, couples in many legal jurisdictions are free to choose to terminate a pregnancy on any grounds in practice. Amniocentesis at about 14 weeks provides similar information and choice. Serum screening detects markers of fetal status in the maternal blood. Ultrasound at 11 and 20 weeks gestation is frequently performed providing fine anatomical detail of the fetus, including sex.
>
> PGD [preimplantation genetic diagnosis] provides an alternative which does not require abortion. It requires IVF and single sperm injection (Savulescu and Kahane 2009, 275).

DeGrazia (2012), in his discussion of prenatal genetic interventions, does indicate that the fact that such interventions require IVF, which "tends to be highly taxing and uncomfortable for women" (99), presents a limitation to their use. But he fails to explore the consequences of the need for IVF in his defense of the use of reprogenetic technologies. Moreover, he believes that advances such as egg and tissue cryopreservation might make the use of IVF "more attractive to many women" (100), neglecting the fact that in order for eggs to be cryopreserved, women must first provide them. He does, however, focus extensively on the moral status of fetuses and embryos.[1] Similarly, when discussing procreative liberty and the right to use reprogenetic technologies, Robertson usually refers to "couples" in his work (e.g. Robertson 1994, 1996, 2003). However, he often mentions women and points out that they assume greater burdens than men in the use of most reproductive technologies. He concedes that it is necessary to take into account possible harms to women when evaluating the freedom to use these technologies. But, again, no substantial discussion is presented on what these greater burdens are or how such burdens need to be taken into account. And his conclusion is that interference with the use of these technologies is unacceptable despite the prejudice that some uses (e.g., sex selection) may reveal toward women (Robertson 2003, 462). Likewise, when defending genetic enhancement of our offspring, neither Savulescu (2005), nor Harris (2007), nor Buchanan (2011), nor DeGrazia (2012) deals at all with the burdens and risks that such practice would pose to women. In fact, when they consider risks related to the development and implementation of genetic enhancement technologies,

---

1. One migh object that one of the main purposes of DeGrazia's book is to shade light on questions about the moral status of prenatal entities. This is indeed correct. Nonetheless, the explicit purpose of the book is *"to illuminate a cluster of ethical issues connected to human reproduction and human genetics through the lens of moral philosophy."* (DeGrazia 2012, 4, emphasis in original). Clearly, women's roles in human reproduction are certainly relevant, particularly when reproduction involves the use of invasive technologies. Moreover, the creation of embryos and fetuses, requires the involvement of women in different, and morally relevant ways than that of men.

risks to women are rarely mentioned, if at all. More often than not, the debates about these technologies simply stipulate that their use is predicated on their safety and efficacy, disregarding the fact that, whatever other known and unknown risks might result from the development and use of these technologies, they will surely impose well-known risks on women.

Of course, I am not suggesting that it is always inapt to talk about "couples" or "reproducers" when discussing issues related to reproduction. But it is certainly striking that the role of women in reproduction in general, and in the use of reprogenetic technologies in particular, is simply absent from these discussions. After all, even when couples participate in reprogenetic projects and make decisions about these technologies, it is not couples but women who have to undergo the risks and burdens of IVF. Likewise, insofar as the concern is with the selection or genetic manipulation of embryos, the "reproducers'" of relevance are also women.

The absence of any significant discussion about the role of women in the development and implementation of reprogenetics or the risks these technologies pose for women is underscored by the fact that proponents of reprogenetics make a point of addressing criticisms regarding the potential adverse consequences of these technologies. Although such criticisms are often dismissed as insufficient or plainly silly, all of these authors discuss a variety of potential negative impacts of using reprogenetics. For instance, they all address possible harms to embryos and to offspring, concerns about playing god, and threats to human nature. Most of them also attend to the effects of these technologies on people with disabilities (DeGrazia 2012; Harris 2007; Savulescu and Kahane 2009).[2] Some of these issues are given a

---

2. Importantly, although the potential effects of reprogenetics on people thought to be disabled are addressed by most mainstream reprogenetic proponents— even when such discussion is often focused on rejecting criticisms presented by

significant amount of attention. For example, Green (2007) dedicates a whole chapter to discussing the "playing god" argument. Harris (2007) does the same with questions about the moral status of embryos. Buchannan (2011) extensively addresses potential harms to human nature.

Of course, I am not arguing that addressing potential negative consequences to offspring or to people with disabilities is inappropriate. On the contrary, such issues are very much part of what an appropriate evaluation of these technologies should include. Neither am I suggesting that attempts to respond to concerns raised by critics of reprogenetics are beside the point. What I am stressing is that if considerations about the possible adverse impacts of these technologies are relevant, and they certainly are, then failing to examine the effect of these technologies on women, both individually and collectively, constitutes a grave oversight.

Reprogenetic Technologies and Women

Feminist scholars have repeatedly called attention to the fact that scientific knowledge and technological innovations are rarely gender-neutral (see, for instance, Anderson 2004; Haraway 1988; Harding 1986; Keller 1985; Longino 1987; Mahowald 2000; Rolin 2004; Wajcman 2004; Wylie and Nelson 2007). Not only have women been historically excluded from

---

disability scholars—their evaluations are seriously deficient. This is so in part precisely because they fail to take account of the context in which reprogenetic technologies are developed and implemented and also because the beliefs of most proponents regarding disability, quality of life, and well-being are quite misguided (see, for instance, Asch 1999, 2003; Barnes 2014; Garland-Thomson 2012; Goering 2008; Mills 2011; Parens and Asch 1999; Scully 2008; Shakespeare 2006; Tremain 2001; Wasserman and Asch 2006).

professional scientific practices (Burrelli 2008; Butcher 2011; Sheltzer and Smith 2014), but the methods, data, and knowledge of science have frequently been used to justify such exclusion (Code 1991; Haraway 1988; Harding 1991; Schiebinger 1989). Feminist scholars have also shown that the ideal of objectivity itself, as traditionally interpreted, is laden with androcentric values and that scientific theories are plagued with gender biases (Fausto-Sterling 1992; Haraway 1989; Hrdy 1986; Jordan-Young 2010; Lloyd 2005; Spanier 1995). Similarly, feminists have shown that issues of concern to women and other marginalized groups have been routinely sidelined as subjects of scientific inquiry and that the scientific and technological knowledge that is produced is often of little use for those in subordinate positions (Harding 2008; Schiebinger 2004; Wajcman 2004). When matters relevant to women are investigated, they are often treated in ways that reproduce gender-normative stereotypes or serve to reinforce oppressive social hierarchies (Harding 1991; Fausto-Sterling 2000; Martin 1987; Richardson 2012; Tuana 1993).

Moreover, science and technology frequently have differential impacts on men and women. Nowhere is this more obvious than in the case of reproductive science and technology, with the development of contraceptive methods directed mostly at women, research on infertility until very recently focused overwhelmingly on women, and the development of technologies to address infertility using women's bodies even in cases of male infertility (Arditti, Klein, and Minden 1984; Corea 1985; Roberts 1997; Rowland 1992). Indeed, it is no accident that feminists have devoted a significant amount of attention to the gender-laden aspects of reproductive technologies and sciences (Arditti, Klein, and Minden 1984; Callahan 1995; Corea 1987; Donchin 1993; Duden 1993; Mahowald 2000; Martin 1987; Overall 1987; Purdy 1996; Roberts 1997; Rothman 1989; Sherwin 1992). This makes all the more conspicuous both the absence of references to this literature and the absence of these concerns in the works of mainstream proponents of reprogenetic technologies.

Importantly, though, even when often treated as such, genetic sciences and technologies are not any more gender-neutral than reproductive sciences and technologies (Mahowald 2000; Richardson 2012; Spanier 1995). Genetic interventions in particular directly and differentially affect women's bodies and impact women's lives (d'Agincourt-Canning 2006; Mahowald 2000). Take, for instance, carrier testing and screening, which is usually used to give prospective parents information about their genetic status so that they can make educated decisions about reproduction. Carriers are individuals who have one normal and one mutated copy of a gene associated with a disease. Because carriers have a normal copy, they ordinarily do not exhibit symptoms of the genetic disorder. Carriers can, however, transmit the mutated allele to their offspring. If a recessive allele is inherited from both parents, the child can be affected by the disease in question. Recessive traits for which carrier testing is common include cystic fibrosis, Tay-Sachs disease, and sickle cell anemia. Although at first glance the decision to undergo carrier testing for reproductive reasons might seem to affect women and men equally, in actuality this is far from the case. Research on population-based screening programs indicates that women tend to accept offers of free carrier testing for particular genetic conditions (e.g., cystic fibrosis) more often than men do (Bekker et al. 1993; Evans et al. 1997). Women also tend to be tested initially when there might be a risk of transmission of a genetic mutation to a couple's children; only if the woman tests positive for a recessive disorder is the male partner involved in the testing (Mahowald 2000). Some have suggested that this discrepancy might occur because men see carrier testing as related to reproductive choices and thus more of a woman's responsibility (Bekker et al. 1993; d'Agincourt-Canning 2006). It might also be related to the sense of responsibility for and to others that women tend to have. Another factor might be that women tend to use primary health care services more than men (Bertakis et al. 2000). Whatever the reason, it is clear that carrier testing affects men and women unequally.

But if science and technology in general, and reproductive and genetic sciences and technologies in particular, are gendered, then analyzing reprogenetic technologies as if they were gender-neutral is inappropriate for a variety of reasons. First, it offers a mistaken description of these technologies. Although couples might indeed make decisions about whether, when, and what type of technologies to use, only women's bodies are directly involved in the use of IVF. And all of the genetic interventions necessary for selecting and enhancing embryos require the use of IVF. Gender-neutral analyses simply conceal the differential burdens of these technologies on men's and women's bodies. Second, gender-neutral examinations obscure the unequal effects that reproductive decisions have on men's and women's lives. Third, ignoring the gendered aspects of reprogenetics is likely to contribute to injustices against women. In what follows, I discuss these concerns in detail.

It bears repeating that gendered analysis of reprogenetic technologies, or indeed of scientific and technological knowledge and implementation in general, need not presuppose a problematic essentialist view of women. It seems clear that reprogenetic technologies have disparate effects on differently situated women. For instance, in the United States, where access to reprogenetic technologies depends on ability to pay, white, economically well-off women constitute the main users of these technologies (Spar 2006). On the other hand, as the burgeoning market in cross-border reproductive care shows, poor women are often the ones providing eggs and serving as gestational carriers (Dickenson 2011; Donchin 2010; Twine 2015). Whereas white, middle-class women are encouraged to use these technologies, a variety of laws and institutional practices discourage women of color from having children (Roberts 1997). Likewise, the main aim of these technologies is to prevent the birth of children with particular diseases and disabilities, so women who are thought to be at higher risk of having children considered disabled are a target group (Parens and Asch 1999; Scully 2008; Shakespeare 2006; Tremain 2001). Nonetheless, although women in different social positions can be affected by these technologies in very different ways, this does not mean that they do not have anything in common (Roberts 2009). Analysis of the intersectionality of gender with other social categories such as race, disability status, class, and nationality is likely to provide unique insight, but this does not mean that attention to gender is irrelevant (Alcoff 2006; Haslanger 2000; Witt 2011).

Reprogenetic Technologies and Risks to Women's Health

Although, as I have pointed out, one would not know it by reading mainstream defenses of reprogenetic technologies, women's bodies are implicated in the development and implementation of these technologies in very different ways from those of men. The effects of these technologies on men's and women's bodies are also significantly different. This, however, has not prevented Savulescu and Kahane (2009) from discussing the use of IVF thus: "[W]hether *parents* should undergo IVF in order to select the most advantaged child does depend on the costs—financial, emotional and physical" (283, my emphasis). As we saw in chapter 2, parents do not undergo IVF, women do. The involvement of men's bodies in IVF is limited to the provision of sperm, a task that involves few health risks.[3] On the other hand, undergoing IVF presents women with a variety of such risks.

The fertility drugs that women must use to stimulate ovulation can cause various side effects including bloating, abdominal pain, and mood swings. In some cases, they can result in ovarian hyperstimulation syndrome (OHSS), a condition that causes a buildup of fluid in the abdomen and lungs (Nastri et al. 2015). Symptoms of OHSS include abdominal pain, bloating, rapid weight gain, nausea, vomiting, and impaired kidney function. The related dehydration can lead to blood clots to the lungs or other organs that may be life-threatening. Mild cases can usually be treated with bed rest, but more severe cases may require hospitalization. The incidence of moderate to severe OHSS is between 3% and 10% of IVF cycles but can be as high as 20% in high-risk women.

Evidence for whether ovarian stimulation protocols result in an increased risk of gynecological cancers such as ovarian, endometrial, cervical, and breast cancers is ambiguous. Some earlier studies suggested an increased risk of these cancers (Brinton et al. 2005; Rossing et al. 1994; Shushan et al. 1996; Whittemore, Harris, and Itnyre 1992). However, more recent, larger studies and systematic reviews have not found evidence of a link between fertility drugs and gynecological cancers (Asante et al. 2013; Bjornholt et al. 2015; Brinton et al. 2013; Kurta et al. 2012; Rizzuto, Behrens, and Smith 2013; Yli-Kuha et al. 2012; Zhao et al. 2015). Nonetheless, because the majority of the women exposed to these drugs are only now beginning to reach the age

3. I am not claiming that the provision of sperm has no relevant effects on men. Clearly, insofar as this activity is related to infertility problems, providing sperm can produce significant stress and anxiety. My point is simply that the technical aspects related to sperm provision do not present health risks to men.

range for many gynecological cancers, it may still be too early to determine whether any increased cancer risks exists.

Egg retrieval procedures also result in health risks to women, including allergic reactions to the anesthesia used during the surgical procedure, bleeding, infection, and injury to organs near the ovaries, such as the bladder or bowel (Nastri et al. 2015). On rare occasions, bowel or blood vessel damage can require emergency surgery and blood transfusions.

IVF also increases the risk of an ectopic pregnancy (i.e., a pregnancy in which the embryo implants outside the intrauterine cavity). It is not clear what specific factors associated with IVF affect the rate of ectopic pregnancy, but its incidence after IVF is significantly higher than in natural pregnancies. The incidence ranges from 2% to 11% of all clinical pregnancies after IVF, whereas 1% to 2% of pregnancies in the general population are ectopic (Li et al. 2015; Refaat, Dalton, and Ledger 2015). Ectopic pregnancies can result in rupture, leading to internal bleeding, pelvic and abdominal pain, shock, and sometimes death.

A variety of health risks are likewise associated with the multiple pregnancies that usually result from the transfer of more than one embryo (Kissin et al. 2015). Multiple pregnancies in IVF treatments are common, particularly in the United States, where in 2012, for instance, only about 20% of transfers involved one embryo and about 25% involved three or more embryos (CDC, American Society for Reproductive Medicine, and Society for Assisted Reproductive Technology 2014). The rate of multiple pregnancies after IVF in the United States is about 30%, whereas in Europe—where often regulations about the number of embryos that can be transferred are stricter—it is about 19% (ESHRE 2014). Risks to women associated with multiple pregnancies include hemorrhage, miscarriage, pregnancy-related high blood pressure, gestational diabetes, and delivery by cesarean section. Although the risks to women's health associated with multiple pregnancies also occur when such pregnancies are the result of natural conception, some evidence suggests that multiple pregnancies after IVF treatment carry increased risks of premature rupture of membranes, gestational diabetes mellitus, pregnancy-induced hypertension, preterm birth, low birth weight, and congenital malformation, compared with those conceived naturally (Qin et al. 2015).

Multiple births also have negative effects on the babies, particularly because of prematurity. Premature babies are at higher risk for a variety of health complications such as low birth weight, perinatal death, psychomotor impairment, lung development problems, intestinal infections, and cerebral palsy (Murray and Norman 2014). Similarly, risks of congenital anomalies are 27% higher in multiple pregnancies than in singleton pregnancies (Boyle et al. 2013). Because women are usually children's' primary caretakers, the birth of multiple babies also has a significant effect on women's physical and psychosocial well-being. Mothers of multiples report lower quality of life and decreased marital satisfaction; they are also at elevated risk for mental health problems such as depression and for parenting stress (Ellison et al. 2005; Roca-de Bes, Gutierrez-Maldonado, and Gris-Martínez 2011).

But reprogenetic technologies present risks also to women who provide the eggs for other women, not simply to those who undergo IVF. Egg providers, as we saw in chapter 2, also have to undergo injections with fertility drugs, and thus they are at risk for the side effects associated with hormonal medications. These risks affect not only women who donate eggs for reproductive purposes but also those who provide eggs for research. This constitutes another significant oversight in current defenses of reprogenetic technologies. After all, the development of these technologies requires research on embryos, necessitating access to eggs. Although some of this research can be done on embryos left over from fertility treatments, at least some of it requires newly donated eggs. For instance, research that has been done to evaluate the feasibility of mitochondrial transfer in human beings involved the use of freshly harvested oocytes (Craven et al. 2010; Paull et al. 2013; Tachibana et al. 2013). In one study (Paull et al. 2013), four women donated 62 oocytes. In another (Tachibana et al. 2013), 106 oocytes were obtained from seven women who underwent ovarian stimulation.

Reproductive Decisions and Women's Lives

Reprogenetic technologies do not simply affect men's and women's bodies in ways that are more burdensome and risky for women. Decisions tied to the use of these technologies also have morally relevant differential effects on men and women, and these also overburden women. Although proponents of reprogenetics often use the rhetoric of choice to defend these technologies, their gender-neutral analysis betrays a disregard for the ways in which the presumed "increase in individual choice" can actually contribute to restricting the choices of many individual women and can affect women's status.

Reprogenetic enthusiasts such as Harris, Savulescu, Robertson, Buchanan, Agar, Silver, and DeGrazia attempt to distinguish their eugenic sympathies from the "old eugenics" precisely by insisting on individual choice. Under the assumption that the problematic aspects of the eugenics programs of the early 20th century were the result of government interference, the liberal eugenics that they embrace condemns authoritarian state impositions and endorses the primacy of the individual in making reprogenetic decisions. Additionally, for these authors, whereas the old eugenics was concerned with improving society's gene pool, liberal eugenics focuses on individual parents' desire to care about the genes of their own children. In Savulescu's words:

What was objectionable about the eugenics movement, besides its shoddy scientific basis, was that it involved the imposition of a state vision for a healthy population and aimed to achieve this through coercion. The eugenics movement was not aimed at what was good for individuals, but rather at what benefited society (Savulescu 2005, 38).

Similarly, Agar (2005), a prominent proponent of liberal eugenics, embraces its goals while distinguishing it from the "old" eugenic programs. He says:

> [S]witching attention from races and classes of humans to individuals provides a version of eugenics worthy of defence. We would be rejecting *authoritarian eugenics*, the idea that the state should have sole responsibility for determining what counts as a good human life, in favour of what I will call *liberal eugenics*. On the liberal approach to human improvement, the state would not presume to make any eugenic choices. Rather it would foster the development of a wide range of technologies of enhancement ensuring that prospective parents were fully informed about what kinds of people these technologies would make. Parents' particular conceptions of the good life would guide them in their selection of enhancements for their children (Agar 2005, 5, emphasis in original).

For advocates of reprogenetics, then, state neutrality is paramount, with governments having at most the role of facilitating individuals' choices. Individuals in general and prospective parents in particular are free to use reprogenetic technologies in whatever way they see fit, provided that their choices do not harm others. Although these authors do not oppose all regulation (e.g., the state has a role in ensuring the reasonable safety and efficacy of these technologies), their view is that, in general, a free market offers sufficient protections so that individuals can choose to use these technologies according to their own values.

Although this interpretation of the evils of eugenic programs is, in my view, rightly contested (Paul 2014) and ignores the tensions between proponents of reprogenetics' liberal tendencies and their eugenic ones (Sparrow 2011), my concern here focuses on the gendered nature of liberal eugenic proposals used to defend reprogenetic technologies and, hence, their effects on women. First, the assumption that these technologies provide women with more choices and that this is a valuable benefit ignores the costs that result from increased choices (Dworkin 1982; Schwartz 2004; Velleman 1992). One such cost is that of acquiring information in order to choose appropriately. The development and introduction of whole genome sequencing technologies make these costs more significant because unparalleled amounts of genetic information can be generated about an individual (Reuter, Spacek, and Snyder 2015). This point is even more salient in the context of reprogenetic technologies because they do more than simply allow women to have offspring with or without particular traits; they permit a choice *among* candidates. Given the increasing amount of information that genetic techniques can provide, decision-making costs are not irrelevant. We saw in chapter 4 the difficulties prospective parents are likely to have when selecting among embryos, all of which have multiple traits, both desirable and undesirable. The more information that can be gathered about the genomic endowment of embryos, the more difficult, and thus more costly, will be the decision. Insofar as reprogenetic technologies are promoted as increasing *women's* choices, the costs of decision making also accrue to women.

Second, the presumption that more choice is better than less choice neglects the relevance of the social and political context in which those choices are presented, the ways in which the framing of those choices affects who can choose or what can be chosen, how social and political factors condition choice, and the constraints that new choices introduce. The concern about the valuation of choice is a version of a general critique of liberalism that often abstracts the individual from relations of power and her choices from the context in which they are made (Schwartzman 2006).

For these reasons, the concept of a gender-neutral individual choice obscures the effects that new technological options have on women in general and also on particular women. It conceals the fact that women, and only women, get pregnant and that only women have to run the health risks associated with choosing to use these technologies. It also neglects the fact that women's reproductive decisions are continuously scrutinized, particularly the decisions of women who do not fit the normative understanding of the good mother, such as poor women, women of color, and women considered to have some disability (Asch 1999; Ettorre 2002; Kleege 2006; Roberts 1997). Women's decisions about whether to get pregnant, when to do so, and how to manage their pregnancy are open to inspection. Pregnant women must control what they put into their bodies, sacrifice their pleasures and desires in order to limit even the slightest of risks to their fetuses, and submit to expert medical knowledge (Duden 1993; Ettorre 2002; Kukla 2005). Indeed, as evidence shows, many women feel they have little choice to say "no" when prenatal genetic testing is recommended by health care professionals (d'Agincourt-Canning 2006; Mahowald 2000). With their simplistic notion of choice, proponents of reprogenetic technologies fail to pay attention to the ways in which, by bringing about some choices, technological interventions also make other choices more difficult or impossible. Of course, these effects of increased choice can affect everyone and not just women, but because reproductive decisions are thought to be the responsibility of women, constraints on some choices (e.g., deciding not to have genetic testing) and the opening of others (e.g., deciding not to have a child who will be thought disabled) are of particular relevance to women.

Third, in ignoring the gendered nature of reproductive choices, proponents of reprogenetics fail to give due attention to the fact that women already tend to see themselves as responsible for the well-being of family members. This is, in part, the result of many women's understanding of the self.[4] They tend to see the self not as an atomized, autonomous agent but as constructed in relation to others, as an interdependent self (Donchin 2001; Mackenzie and Stoljar 1999; McLeod 2002; Sherwin 1992). They are more likely to see their lives as interconnected with the lives of others and to define themselves in term of their social relationships with others and their obligations to them. In this context, the availability of reprogenetic technologies—technologies that are presented as aiming to bring into the world children with the most expected well-being—are bound to have a more burdensome effect on women than on men. Women already seem to be prepared to undergo potentially risky medical interventions to fulfill their perceived obligation of caring for others (Hallowell 1999; McCabe and McCabe 2011). Moreover, women who are identified as being at risk of suffering some genetic condition that they could pass on to their children also assume responsibility for managing such risks. Of course, casting the use of these technologies as a moral obligation is even more troublesome. As indicated, Savulescu and Kahane (2009) explicitly advocate that

---

4. This, again, does not involve a problematic essentialism. Women's conceptions of the self need not be grounded on some essential property of womanhood—or manhood, for that matter—but are formed in relation to the social positions that women occupy.

women undertake the risks of IVF in order to maximize the well-being of their future children. In their own words:

> [A]lthough women should not undergo risky fertility treatments in order to be able to select an embryo whose expected well-being is only negligibly greater than that of the child they expect to have naturally, we believe that PB instructs women to seriously consider IVF if natural reproduction is likely to lead to a child with a condition that is expected to reduce well-being significantly, even if that condition is not a disease (281).

Fourth, presenting reproductive choices related to reprogenetics as gender-neutral also disregards the relationships among choice, responsibility, and blame. Once one is aware that a particular choice is available (e.g., to use PGD to select against embryos with undesirable characteristics), the failure to choose counts against one; one is now responsible, and can be held responsible, for the choice in question (Dworkin 1982). Insofar as these technologies are available, and more so if their use is thought to present a moral obligation, women can both blame themselves and be blamed by others for the choices they make. Whereas before the advent of these technologies women could not be thought of as blameworthy for choosing to bring a child into the world who was judged less than the best, now they can.[5] Surely, as proponents of reprogenetics like to point out, to not use these technologies is also to make a choice—a choice to, as they contend,

---

5. Of course, women have, and still are, often blamed for creating children with what are thought to be undesirable traits (see discussion below for more on this). But blaming women for the ill health of their children is different than blaiming them for *choosing to bring* such children into the world when they could have done otherwise. Before technologies that permitted such choosing were available, women could not be blamed. Now they can.

let the randomness of the natural lottery act. But that is just the point: Women can now be held and hold themselves responsible for using or failing to use these technologies. They can also be held and hold themselves responsible for the particular embryo they happen to select. They can now reasonably be asked to justify their choice of *this* child. Insofar as the child in question is thought to have undesirable characteristics that could have been eliminated by selecting a different embryo, such justification will be necessary to avoid blame. Moreover, both disability and disease are thought by proponents of reprogenetic technologies to decrease well-being and are thus considered targets for these technologies. The decisions of women who are thought to be at risk of having children with such characteristics would therefore be particularly scrutinized, and their choices, especially when they do not conform to societal expectations, would require justification.

Of course, to claim that introducing new reproductive choices can have negative costs, particularly for women, is not to argue that it is always better to have fewer choices. In many contexts, having increased choices promotes well-being, and to that extent, choices are valuable. However, that costs of increased choice exist, that they affect women and men in very different ways that tend to be disadvantageous for women, and that they have negative impacts on women's lives are reasons not simply to attend to these costs but to do so in a way that recognizes the gendered nature of reproductive decisions.

Likewise, the fact that the obligations to select and enhance one's offspring impose more burdens on women is not by itself a problem. After all, role obligations attach to people in particular social roles. People have particular obligations that stem from their roles as parents, teachers, government officials, doctors, midwives, gardeners, and so on. Meeting these duties can place different burdens on an individual, and this need not be unjust or unfair. Hence, the idea that women have obligations that emanate from their reproductive capacities and their roles as mothers or caregivers seems, at least in principle, unproblematic. Nonetheless, the concerns discussed earlier are the result of constructing women's social roles related to reproduction in ways that systematically disadvantage them. Nothing about the social roles that men and women occupy requires that women be thought of as more responsible for reproductive decisions than men. True, differential burdens on men and women will result from the fact that only women get pregnant and give birth. But insofar as this is so, attention must be given to social practices and norms that can make the fulfilling of one's duties more or less onerous or that can either assist people in meeting their obligations or obstruct their ability to do so. Moreover, that obligations to use reprogenetic technologies affect women and men differentially, and that they affect women negatively, is certainly a reason to acknowledge these facts rather than to treat the effects of these obligations and choices in a gender-neutral way.

Injustices against Women

Ignoring the ways in which the gendered nature of reprogenetic choices have differential impacts on women's health and decisions is problematic because it misrepresents the real effects of reprogenetic technologies. In this way, mainstream evaluations of these technologies are simply misleading. Such neglect is also suspect because it is likely to increase injustices against women. This is so for several reasons. First, gender-neutral defenses of reprogenetic technologies disregard the ways in which the actual development and implementation of these technologies can contribute to overburdening women. Recall that the explicit aim of reprogenetic technologies is to create "better" babies. This is likely to expand the already extensive surveillance and control of women's choices regarding reproduction. Women's decisions regarding whether to become pregnant, when to do so, and what to do during pregnancy are open to criticism. Even choices that might appear insignificant at any other time acquire oversized roles when women are pregnant or are considering becoming pregnant. Pregnant women are strongly, and anxiously, advised to take folic acid, to exercise regularly but not excessively, and to avoid alcohol, tobacco, caffeine, unpasteurized milk, and X-rays. They are encouraged—sometimes strongly so when they are thought to belong to an "at risk" category (e.g., more than 35 years old) or to be at risk of transmitting diseases or disabilities—to have prenatal screening to check for fetal abnormalities. They are instructed to breastfeed their newborn so as to create appropriate bonds with the child and ensure adequate nutrition. Studies purportedly showing the significant effects of women's decisions during pregnancy on the well-being of their children are common. What women do or fail to do in their youth, while pregnant, and after a baby is born are said to have serious, sometimes devastating, consequences on children's nutritional status, risk of obesity, allergies, IQ, learning and developmental delays, and behavioral problems (Cao et al. 2014; Grzeskowiak et al. 2015; Tryggvadottir et al. 2015; von Ehrenstein et al. 2015; Wang et al. 2014). As has been widely discussed in the feminist literature, these norms, which women are expected to internalize, can be oppressive for any woman, but they can be experienced as particularly punishing by less privileged women, who often lack the resources and the life circumstances that would allow them to have this degree of control over their pregnancies (Richardson et al. 2014; Kukla 2005; Roberts 1997).

Biomedical technologies have similarly multiplied the degree of scrutiny that women's reproductive decisions and women's lives undergo. Ultrasound is routinely used in the management of pregnant women, as are screening tests to detect a variety of genetic mutations and variants. The use of caesarian sections has increased all over the world (Liu et al. 2007). And women's decisions about whether to have a child at home have become a matter of public policy (ACOG 2011). Reprogenetic technologies extend this scrutiny of women's reproductive decisions in significant ways. Women will likely be expected to make particular kinds of choices—that is, to use these technologies to select embryos with desirable traits and to discard those embryos with characteristics that are thought to fall outside accepted norms. The degree of control over decisions about what children to bring and not bring into the world that these technologies allow can only serve to expand the surveillance of women's bodies and choices—all in the service of ensuring the well-being of fetuses and future children.

It is not simply that this intense scrutiny of women forces them to make innumerable decisions, many of them of significant moral import, and that it increases their anxieties about pregnancy and intensifies their feelings of responsibility for the well-being of their children. It is also that the use of these technologies in a context in which the health and well-being of fetuses is a priority is seen by health care professionals, women themselves, and members of the public as what good mothers ought to do. Women are thus subject to moral condemnation when their choices do not fit what is expected of them. Reprogenetic technologies now place the genetic makeup and well-being of future children more within the apparent control of individual women's choices and thus also within their responsibility. This is not to say that reprogenetic technologies should be rejected for these reasons alone. Rather, it is to argue that the differential moral implications that these technologies have for women need to be considered and addressed in discussions of reprogenetics.

Moreover, the fact that development of at least some reprogenetic technologies requires a supply of eggs in order to perform appropriate research raises questions of exploitation, both nationally and particularly internationally, of the women who will be providing those eggs. In a context of mounting commercialization of eggs and other reproductive services, global poverty, and gender oppression, the development and implementation of reprogenetic technologies is likely to contribute to the exploitation of women in vulnerable situations (Almeling 2011; Dickenson 2011; Donchin 2010). Payment for eggs is becoming more common and more widely accepted, underscoring this concern. Moreover, providers of eggs for research often lack the protections of other human subjects (Magnus and Cho 2005). Egg providers, like human subjects in clinical research, are exposing themselves to sometimes serious risk for the benefit of others. For other research subjects, significant scrutiny and regulatory protections exist because the risks to which they are exposed are related to the research that is being done. In the case of egg providers, however, there is generally nothing experimental about the stimulation and extraction of eggs. Moreover, those involved in obtaining the eggs and those involved in doing the research are usually different professionals. The research happens after the eggs have been obtained, and the protections for egg providers at that stage are usually limited to assurances that informed consent has been obtained, a consent that evidence shows requires significant improvements (Cattapan 2016). Research with anonymized tissue does not usually constitute research with human subjects and therefore does not receive the kind of scrutiny that the latter involves. Although practices for ensuring the informed consent of women providing eggs might be subjected to a degree of control and examination in industrialized nations, global markets for eggs are likely to make such control more difficult.

Second, mainstream gender-neutral assessments of reprogenetic technologies that simply focus on the ways in which these technologies appear to increase choices are implicitly and uncritically sanctioning the status quo. Not only do they fail to draw attention to the social conditions and institutions that systematically disadvantage women, but they also fail to challenge those conditions or offer constructive solutions to them. In ignoring the ways in which women's bodies and decisions are already subjected to intense public scrutiny and censure, proponents of reprogenetic technologies have failed to appreciate how reprogenetics contributes to and increases this scrutiny. At the least, attention to such issues could have resulted in a tempering of the enthusiasm for these technologies.

But proper attention to the effects of reprogenetic technologies on women does not simply lead to a questioning of the fervor that proponents express. Even if one were to accept that the extensive use of selection and enhancement techniques can contribute to societal improvement, acknowledgment of the negative impact of these technologies in women's lives would likely lead to a more appropriate implementation of reprogenetics. For instance, in spite of the growing use of egg providers both for reproductive and research purposes, little attention has been given to the long-term health risks of fertility drugs (Woodriff, Sauer, and Klitzman 2014). Development of reprogenetic technologies aimed at enhancement of embryos is likely to increase the need for women to provide eggs (Dickenson 2013). Attention to the gendered nature of these technologies thus would emphasize the necessity of careful collection and analysis of data on egg providers, the importance of national egg and embryo donor registries, and the need for long-term studies and long-term follow-up. Defenses of reprogenetic technologies that address the well-being of women would underscore not simply the moral obligation to use these technologies but the obligation of relevant institutions (e.g., federal and local governments, health care professionals, biomedical researchers) to ensure that adequate means are used to investigate risks to women's health and to limit such risks.

Likewise, in disregarding the potential for exploitation that can follow from the development of at least some reprogenetic technologies, proponents have missed the opportunity not only to call attention to this possibility but to demand that appropriate mechanisms be put in place to eliminate or reduce these dangers. The lack of consistency in national regulations, the differences in economic incentives among various countries, and pronatalist ideologies all contribute to a context in which egg providers are more likely to be harmed by exploitation. And of course, in neglecting the potential for exploitation of reprogenetic technologies, proponents have failed to call attention or offer solutions to the situational and pathological vulnerabilities to which many women in the world are exposed, vulnerabilities that limit their options and can coerce them into providing eggs for research.

Exploitation is not the only concern raised by the market for human eggs. Ensuring that women are appropriately informed about the risks of drugs that stimulate the ovaries and other physical and psychological consequences of providing eggs is similarly critical. Indeed, given that increased choice is accompanied by increased responsibility (i.e., to choose wisely), the need to ensure that women have adequate information about their choices imposes obligations on clinicians and researchers to produce and make such information available.

Moreover, it is well known that access to suitable prenatal care contributes to the well-being of women and their children. Nonetheless, in 2009–2010 in the United States, more than 17% of recent mothers reported that they were not able to access prenatal care as early as they had wanted (DHHS and HRSA 2013). Women of color report being particularly affected by such lack of access. Unsurprisingly, one of the most common barriers to getting prenatal care at all or as early as desired is limited resources. Worldwide, inadequate attention to pregnancy and childbirth claimed the lives of 303,000 women in 2015, and most of these deaths could have been prevented (WHO 2015). Furthermore, 2.7 million babies die every year in their first month of life, at least in part because their mothers did not have access to adequate prenatal health care and nutrition (WHO 2016). An interest in helping women to manage possible risks to the well-being of their future children (a presumed goal of the development of reprogenetics), one that is attentive to the ways in which women's reproductive decisions can be constrained, will surely lead proponents of reprogenetic technologies to forcefully and heartily defend the need for adequate access to integrated and flexible prenatal services.

Conclusion

In Shakespeare's play *Macbeth*, the three wiches assure Macbeth that "none of woman born" will harm him (Act 4, Scene 1). Had he been a believer in the mainstream defenses of reprogenetics, Macbeth would have been easily convinced that he had nothing to fear because he would have thought that women had nothing to do with the birth of children. In their enthusiasm for the individual and social benefits that reprogenetic technologies will presumably confer, advocates have overlooked the crucial role of women in the development and implementation of these technologies and their effects on women's lives. That women are the ones who must undergo IVF with its associated risks, the ones who get pregnant, and the ones who are often held responsible for reproductive decisions seems to be of no relevance to proponents of these technologies. Their concern with expanding reproductive choices appears to have clouded their ability to reflect on the ways in which the social and political context affects who can choose or what can be chosen, as well as what are thought to be appropriate or inappropriate choices and the ways in which choices are not simply expanded but also constrained. Equally troubling, in erasing women from their assessments, advocates of reprogenetics have failed to recognize how these technologies can contribute to furthering injustices against women and have missed the opportunity to draw our attention to the structural problems that must be transformed to avoid such injustices. Whether or not Macbeth could have avoided his fate by realizing that even those who appear to be "not of woman born" in fact are so born, it seems clear that any evaluation of reprogenetic technologies that ignores women fails to provide an ethically sound assessment of these technologies.

References

(ACOG) American Congress of Obstetricians and Gynecologists, Committee on Obstetric Practice. 2011. ACOG committee opinion no. 476: planned home birth. *Obstetrics and Gynecology* 117 (2 Part 1):425–8. http://www.ncbi.nlm.nih.gov/pubmed/21252776.

Agar, Nicholas. 2005. *Liberal eugenics: in defence of human enhancement.* Malden, MA: Blackwell Publishing.

Alcoff, Linda. 2006. *Visible identities: race, gender, and the self.* Studies in Feminist Philosophy. New York: Oxford University Press.

Almeling, Rene. 2011. *Sex cells: the medical market for eggs and sperm.* Berkeley: University of California Press.

Anderson, Elizabeth. 2004. Uses of value judgments in science: a general argument, with lessons from a case study of feminist research on divorce. *Hypatia* 19 (1):1–24.

Arditti, Rita, Renate Klein, and Shelley Minden. 1984. *Test-tube women: what future for motherhood?* Boston: Pandora Press.

Asante, A., P. H. Leonard, A. L. Weaver, E. L. Goode, J. R. Jensen, E. A. Stewart, and C. C. Coddington. 2013. Fertility drug use and the risk of ovarian tumors in infertile women: a case-control study. *Fertility and Sterility* 99 (7):2031–6.

Asch, Adrienne. 1999. Prenatal diagnosis and selective abortion: a challenge to practice and policy. *American Journal of Public Health* 89 (11):1649–57.

———. 2003. Disability equality and prenatal testing: contradictory or compatible? *Florida State University Law Review* 30 (2):315–42.

Barnes, Elizabeth. 2014. Valuing disability, causing disability. *Ethics* 125 (1):88–113.

Bekker, H., M. Modell, G. Denniss, A. Silver, C. Mathew, M. Bobrow, and T. Marteau. 1993. Uptake of cystic fibrosis testing in primary care: supply push or demand pull? *BMJ* 306 (6892):1584–6.

Bertakis, K. D., R. Azari, L. J. Helms, E. J. Callahan, and J. A. Robbins. 2000. Gender differences in the utilization of health care services. *Journal of Family Practice* 49 (2):147–52.

Bjornholt, Sarah Marie, Susanne Kruger Kjaer, Thor Schutt Svane Nielsen, and Allan Jensen. 2015. Risk for borderline ovarian tumours after exposure to fertility drugs: results of a population-based cohort study. *Human Reproduction* 30 (1):222–31.

Boyle, B., R. McConkey, E. Garne, et al. 2013. Trends in the prevalence, risk and pregnancy outcome of multiple births with congenital anomaly: a registry-based study in 14 European countries 1984–2007. *BJOG* 120 (6):707–16.

Brinton, L. A., K. S. Moghissi, B. Scoccia, C. L. Westhoff, and E. J. Lamb. 2005. Ovulation induction and cancer risk. *Fertility and Sterility* 83 (2):261–74.

Brinton, L. A., Britton Trabert, Varda Shalev, Eitan Lunenfeld, Tal Sella, and Gabriel Chodick. 2013. In vitro fertilization and risk of breast and gynecologic cancers: a retrospective cohort study within the Israeli Maccabi Healthcare Services. *Fertility and Sterility* 99 (5):1189–1196.

Buchanan, Allen E. 2011. *Beyond humanity?: the ethics of biomedical enhancement*. New York: Oxford University Press.

Burrelli, J. 2008. Thirty-three years of women in S&E faculty positions. Washington, DC: National Science Foundation.

Butcher, J. 2011. Women in science and medicine. *Lancet* 377 (9768):811–2.

Callahan, Joan C. 1995. *Reproduction, ethics, and the law: feminist perspectives*. Bloomington, IN: Indiana University Press.

Cao, B., M. J. Stout, I. Lee, and I. U. Mysorekar. 2014. Placental microbiome and its role in preterm birth. *Neoreviews* 15 (12):e537–45.

Cattapan, A.R. 2016. Good eggs? Evaluating consent forms for egg donation. *Journal of Medical Ethics*.

(CDC) Centers for Disease Control and Prevention, American Society for Reproductive Medicine, and Society for Assisted Reproductive Technology. 2014. *2012 Assisted reproductive technology national summary report*. Atlanta: US Department of Health and Human Services.

Code, Lorraine. 1991. *What can she know?: feminist theory and the construction of knowledge*. Ithaca, NY: Cornell University Press.

Corea, Gena. 1985. *The mother machine: reproductive technologies from artificial insemination to artificial wombs*. 1st ed. New York: Harper & Row.

———. 1987. *Man-made women: how new reproductive technologies affect women*. 1st Midland Book ed. Bloomington, IN: Indiana University Press.

Craven, Lyndsey, Helen A. Tuppen, Gareth D. Greggains, et al. 2010. Pronuclear transfer in human embryos to prevent transmission of mitochondrial DNA disease. *Nature* 465 (7294):82–5.

d'Agincourt-Canning, L. 2006. Genetic testing for hereditary breast and ovarian cancer: responsibility and choice. *Qualitative Health Research* 16 (1):97–118.

DeGrazia, David. 2012. *Creation ethics: reproduction, genetics, and quality of life*. New York: Oxford University Press.

(DHHS) US Department of Health and Human Services, Health Resources and Services Administration, and Health Resources and Services Administration (HRSA), Maternal and Child Health Bureau. 2013. *Child Health USA 2013*. Rockville, MD: DHHS.

Dickenson, Donna. L. 2011. Regulating (or not) reproductive medicine: an alternative to letting the market decide. *Indian Journal of Medical Ethics* 8 (3):175–9.

———. 2013. The commercialization of human eggs in mitochondrial replacement research. *The New Bioethics* 19 (1):18–29.

Donchin, Anne. 1993. *Procreation, power and subjectivity: feminist approaches to new reproductive technologies*. Working Paper Series. Wellesley, MA: Center for Research on Women.

———. 2001. Understanding autonomy relationally: toward a reconfiguration of bioethical principles. *Journal of Medical Philosophy* 26 (4):365–86.

———. 2010. Reproductive tourism and the quest for global gender justice. *Bioethics* 24 (7):323–32.

Duden, Barbara. 1993. *Disembodying women: perspectives on pregnancy and the unborn.* Cambridge, MA: Harvard University Press.

Dworkin, Gerald. 1982. Is more choice better than less? *Midwest Studies in Philosophy* 7 (1):47–61.

Ellison, M. A., S. Hotamisligil, H. Lee, J. W. Rich-Edwards, S. C. Pang, and J. E. Hall. 2005. Psychosocial risks associated with multiple births resulting from assisted reproduction. *Fertility and Sterility* 83 (5):1422–8.

(ESHRE) European Society of Human Reproduction and Embryology. 2014. ART fact sheet. https://www.eshre.eu/Guidelines-and-Legal/ART-fact-sheet.aspx.

Ettorre, Elizabeth. 2002. *Reproductive genetics, gender, and the body.* New York: Routledge.

Evans, D. G., E. R. Maher, R. Macleod, D. R. Davies, and D. Craufurd. 1997. Uptake of genetic testing for cancer predisposition. *Journal of Medical Genetics* 34 (9):746–8.

Fausto-Sterling, Anne. 1992. *Myths of gender: biological theories about women and men.* 2nd ed. New York: BasicBooks.

———. 2000. *Sexing the body: gender politics and the construction of sexuality.* New York: BasicBooks.

Garland-Thomson, Rosemary. 2012. The case for conserving disability. *Journal of Bioethical Inquiry* 9 (3):339–55.

Goering, Sara. 2008. 'You say you're happy, but . . .': contested quality of life judgments in bioethics and disability studies. *Journal of Bioethical Inquiry* 5 (2–3):125–35.

Green, Ronald Michael. 2007. *Babies by design: the ethics of genetic choice.* New Haven, CT: Yale University Press.

Grzeskowiak, L. E., N. A. Hodyl, M. J. Stark, J. L. Morrison, and V. L. Clifton. 2015. Association of early and late maternal smoking during pregnancy with offspring body mass index at 4 to 5 years of age. *Journal of Developmental Origins of Health and Disease* 6 (6):485–92.

Hallowell, N. 1999. Doing the right thing: genetic risk and responsibility. *Sociology of Health and Illness* 21 (5):597–621.

Haraway, Donna. 1988. Situated knowledges: the science question in feminism and the privilege of partial perspective. *Feminist Studies* 14 (3):575–99.

————. 1989. *Primate visions: gender, race, and nature in the world of modern science*. New York: Routledge.

Harding, Sandra G. 1986. *The science question in feminism*. Ithaca, NY: Cornell University Press.

————. 1991. *Whose science? whose knowledge?: thinking from women's lives*. Ithaca, NY: Cornell University Press.

————. 2008. Sciences from below: feminisms, postcolonialities, and modernities. In *Next wave: new directions in women's studies*. Durham, NC: Duke University Press.

Harris, John. 2007. *Enhancing evolution: the ethical case for making better people*. Princeton, NJ: Princeton University Press.

Haslanger, Sally. 2000. Gender and race: (what) are they? (what) do we want them to be? *Noûs* 34 (1):31–55.

Hrdy, Sarah B. 1986. Empathy, polyandry and the myth of the coy female. In *Feminist Approaches to Science*, edited by R. Bleier. New York: Pergamon.

Jordan-Young, Rebecca M. 2010. *Brain storm: the flaws in the science of sex differences*. Cambridge, MA: Harvard University Press.

Keller, Evelyn Fox. 1985. *Reflections on gender and science*. New Haven, CT: Yale University Press.

Kissin, D. M., A. D. Kulkarni, A. Mneimneh, L. Warner, S. L. Boulet, S. Crawford, D. J. Jamieson, and National ART Surveillance System (NASS) Group. 2015. Embryo transfer practices and multiple births resulting from assisted reproductive technology: an opportunity for prevention. *Fertility and Sterility* 103 (4):954–61.

Kleege, Georgina. 2006. *Blind rage: letters to Helen Keller*. Washington, DC: Gallaudet University Press.

Kukla, Rebecca. 2005. *Mass hysteria: medicine, culture, and mothers' bodies*. Explorations in Bioethics and the Medical Humanities. Lanham, MD: Rowman & Littlefield.

Kurta, Michelle L., Kirsten B. Moysich, Joel L. Weissfeld, Ada O. Youk, Clareann H. Bunker, Robert P. Edwards, Francesmary Modugno, Roberta B. Ness, and Brenda Diergaarde. 2012. Use of fertility drugs and risk of ovarian cancer: results from a U.S.-based case-control study. *Cancer Epidemiology Biomarkers and Prevention* 21 (8):1282–92.

Li, Z., E. A. Sullivan, M. Chapman, C. Farquhar, and Y. A. Wang. 2015. Risk of ectopic pregnancy lowest with transfer of single frozen blastocyst. *Human Reproduction* 30 (9):2048–54.

Liu, S., R. M. Liston, K. S. Joseph, M. Heaman, R. Sauve, M. S. Kramer, and Maternal Health Study Group of the Canadian Perinatal Surveillance System. 2007. Maternal mortality and severe morbidity associated with low-risk planned cesarean delivery versus planned vaginal delivery at term. *CMAJ* 176 (4):455–60.

Lloyd, Elisabeth Anne. 2005. *The case of the female orgasm: bias in the science of evolution*. Cambridge, MA: Harvard University Press.

Longino, Helen E. 1987. Can there be a feminist science? *Hypatia* 2 (3):51–64.

Mackenzie, Catriona, and Natalie Stoljar. 1999. *Relational autonomy: feminist perspectives on autonomy, agency, and the social self.* New York: Oxford University Press.

Magnus, D., and M. K. Cho. 2005. Ethics: issues in oocyte donation for stem cell research. *Science* 308 (5729):1747–8.

Mahowald, Mary Briody. 2000. *Genes, women, equality*. New York: Oxford University Press.

Martin, Emily. 1987. *The woman in the body: a cultural analysis of reproduction*. Boston: Beacon Press.

McCabe, L. L., and E. R. McCabe. 2011. Down syndrome: coercion and eugenics. *Genetics in Medicine* 13 (8):708–10.

McLeod, Carolyn. 2002. *Self-trust and reproductive autonomy*. Basic Bioethics. Cambridge, MA: MIT Press.

Mills, Catherine. 2011. The limits of reproductive autonomy: prenatal testing, harm and disability. *Futures of Reproduction: Bioethics and Biopolitics* 49:57–83.

Murray, S. R., and J. E. Norman. 2014. Multiple pregnancies following assisted reproductive technologies: a happy consequence or double trouble? *Seminars in Fetal and Neonatal Medicine* 19 (4):222–7.

Nastri, C. O., D. M. Teixeira, R. M. Moroni, V. M. S. Leitao, and W. P. Martins. 2015. Ovarian hyperstimulation syndrome: pathophysiology, staging, prediction and prevention. *Ultrasound in Obstetrics and Gynecology* 45 (4):377–93.

Overall, Christine. 1987. *Ethics and human reproduction: a feminist analysis*. Boston: Allen & Unwin.

Parens, Erik, and Adrienne Asch. 1999. The disability rights critique of prenatal genetic testing: reflections and recommendations. *Hastings Center Report* 29 (5).

Paul, Diane B. 2014. What was wrong with eugenics?: conflicting narratives and disputed interpretations. *Science and Education* 23 (2):259–71.

Paull, Daniel, Valentina Emmanuele, Keren A. Weiss, et al. 2013. Nuclear genome transfer in human oocytes eliminates mitochondrial DNA variants. *Nature* 493 (7434):632–7.

Purdy, Laura M. 1996. *Reproducing persons: issues in feminist bioethics.* Ithaca, NY: Cornell University Press.

Qin, J., H. Wang, X. Sheng, D. Liang, H. Tan, and J. Xia. 2015. Pregnancy-related complications and adverse pregnancy outcomes in multiple pregnancies resulting from assisted reproductive technology: a meta-analysis of cohort studies. *Fertility and Sterility* 103 (6):1492–508.e1–7.

Refaat, B., E. Dalton, and W. L. Ledger. 2015. Ectopic pregnancy secondary to in vitro fertilisation–embryo transfer: pathogenic mechanisms and management strategies. *Reproductive Biology and Endocrinology* 13:30.

Reuter, J. A., D. V. Spacek, and M. P. Snyder. 2015. High-throughput sequencing technologies. *Molecules and Cells* 58 (4):586–97.

Richardson, Sarah. 2012. Sexing the X: how the X became the 'female chromosome.' *Signs* 37 (4):909–33.

Richardson, S., C.R. Daniels, M.W. Gillman, J. Golden, R. Kukla, C. Kuzawa, and J. Rich-Edwards. 2014. Society: Don't blame the mothers. *Nature.* 512(7513):131–2.

Rizzuto, Ivana, Renee F. Behrens, and Lesley A. Smith. 2013. Risk of ovarian cancer in women treated with ovarian stimulating drugs for infertility. *Cochrane Database of Systematic Reviews* 8:CD008215.

Roberts, Dorothy E. 1997. *Killing the black body: race, reproduction, and the meaning of liberty.* New York: Pantheon Books.

———. 2009. Race, gender, and genetic technologies: a new reproductive dystopia? *Signs* 34 (4):783–804.

Robertson, John A. 1994. *Children of choice: freedom and the new reproductive technologies.* Princeton, NJ: Princeton University Press.

———. 1996. Genetic selection of offspring characteristics. *Boston University Law Review* 76 (3):421–82.

———. 2003. Procreative liberty in the era of genomics. *American Journal of Law and Medicine* 29 (4):439–87.

Roca-de Bes, M., J. Gutierrez-Maldonado, and J. M. Gris-Martínez. 2011. Comparative study of the psychosocial risks associated with families with multiple births resulting from assisted reproductive technology (ART) and without ART. *Fertility and Sterility* 96 (1):170–4.

Rolin, Kristina. 2004. Why gender is a relevant factor in the social epistemology of scientific inquiry. *Philosophy of Science* 71 (5):880–91.

Rossing, M. A., J. R. Daling, N. S. Weiss, D. E. Moore, and S. G. Self. 1994. Ovarian tumors in a cohort of infertile women. *New England Journal of Medicine* 331 (12):771–6.

Rothman, Barbara Katz. 1989. *Recreating motherhood: ideology and technology in a patriarchal society.* 1st ed. New York: Norton.

Rowland, Robyn. 1992. *Living laboratories: women and reproductive technologies.* Bloomington, IN: Indiana University Press.

Savulescu, Julian 2001. Procreative beneficence: why we should select the best children. *Bioethics* 15 (5–6):413–26.

———. 2005. New breeds of humans: the moral obligation to enhance. *Reproductive Biomedicine Online* 10:36–9.

Savulescu, Julian, and Guy Kahane. 2009. The moral obligation to create children with the best chance of the best life. *Bioethics* 23 (5):274–90.

Schiebinger, Londa L. 1989. *The mind has no sex?: women in the origins of modern science.* Cambridge, MA: Harvard University Press.

———. 2004. *Plants and empire: colonial bioprospecting in the Atlantic world.* Cambridge, MA: Harvard University Press.

Schwartz, Barry. 2004. *The paradox of choice: why more is less.* 1st ed. New York: Ecco.

Schwartzman, Lisa H. 2006. *Challenging liberalism: feminism as political critique.* University Park, PA: Pennsylvania State University Press.

Scully, Jackie Leach. 2008. *Disability bioethics: moral bodies, moral difference.* Feminist Constructions. Lanham, MD: Rowman & Littlefield.

Shakespeare, Tom. 2006. *Disability rights and wrongs.* New York: Routledge.

Sheltzer, J. M., and J. C. Smith. 2014. Elite male faculty in the life sciences employ fewer women. *Proceedings of the National Academy of Sciences U S A* 111 (28):10107–12.

Sherwin, Susan. 1992. *No longer patient: feminist ethics and health care.* Philadelphia: Temple University Press.

Shushan, A., O. Paltiel, J. Iscovich, U. Elchalal, T. Peretz, and J. G. Schenker. 1996. Human menopausal gonadotropin and the risk of epithelial ovarian cancer. *Fertility and Sterility* 65 (1):13–18.

Spanier, Bonnie. 1995. *Im/partial science: gender ideology in molecular biology.* Bloomington, IN: Indiana University Press.

Spar, Debora L. 2006. *The baby business: how money, science, and politics drive the commerce of conception.* Boston: Harvard Business School Press.

Sparrow, Robert 2011. A not-so-new eugenics: Harris and Savulescu on human enhancement. *Hastings Center Report* 41 (1):32–42.

Tachibana, Masahito, Paula Amato, Michelle Sparman, et al. 2013. Towards germline gene therapy of inherited mitochondrial diseases. *Nature* 493 (7434):627–31.

Tremain, Shelley. 2001. On the government of disability. *Social Theory and Practice* 27:617–36.

Tryggvadottir, E. A., H. Medek, B. E. Birgisdottir, R. T. Geirsson, and I. Gunnarsdottir. 2015. Association between healthy maternal dietary pattern and risk for gestational diabetes mellitus. *European Journal of Clinical Nutrition* 70 (2):237–42.

Tuana, Nancy. 1993. *The less noble sex: scientific, religious, and philosophical conceptions of woman's nature.* Bloomington, IN: Indiana University Press.

Twine, France Winddance. 2015. *Outsourcing the womb: race, class and gestational surrogacy in a global market.* 2nd ed. New York: Routledge.

Velleman, J. D. 1992. Against the right to die. *Journal of Medical Philosophy* 17 (6):665–81.

von Ehrenstein, O. S., H. Aralis, M. E. Flores, and B. Ritz. 2015. Fast food consumption in pregnancy and subsequent asthma symptoms in young children. *Pediatric Allergy and Immunology* 26 (6):571–7.

Wajcman, Judy. 2004. *TechnoFeminism.* Malden, MA: Polity.

Wang, P. J., G. A. Morgan, A. W. Hwang, L. C. Chen, and H. F. Liao. 2014. Do maternal interactive behaviors correlate with developmental outcomes and mastery motivation in toddlers with and without motor delay? *Physical Therapy* 94 (12):1744–54.

Wasserman, David, and Adrienne Asch. 2006. The uncertain rationale for prenatal disability screening. *The Virtual Mentor: VM* 8 (1):53–6.

Weissman, A., M. Leong, M. V. Sauer, and Z. Shoham. 2014. Characterizing the practice of oocyte donation: a web-based international survey. *Reproductive Biomedicine Online* 28 (4):443–50.

Whittemore, A. S., R. Harris, and J. Itnyre. 1992. Characteristics relating to ovarian-cancer risk: collaborative analysis of 12 United-States case-control studies. II: Invasive epithelial ovarian cancers in white women. Collaborative Ovarian Cancer Group. *American Journal of Epidemiology* 136 (10):1184–203.

(WHO) World Health Organization. 2015. *Trends in maternal mortality: 1990 to 2015. 2015. Estimates by WHO, UNICEF, UNFPA, World Bank Group and the United Nations Population Division.* Geneva: World Health Organization. http://apps.who.int/iris/bitstream/10665/194254/1/9789241565141_eng.pdf?ua=1

———. 2016. Children: reducing mortality. Fact sheet no. 178. http://www.who.int/mediacentre/factsheets/fs178/en/

Witt, Charlotte. 2011. *The metaphysics of gender.* Studies in Feminist Philosophy. New York: Oxford University Press.

Woodriff, M., M. V. Sauer, and R. Klitzman. 2014. Advocating for longitudinal follow-up of the health and welfare of egg donors. *Fertility and Sterility* 102 (3):662–6.

Wylie, Alison, and Lynn Hankinson Nelson. 2007. Coming to terms with the values of science: insights from feminist science studies scholarship. In *Value-free science?: ideals and illusions*, edited by H. Kincaid, J. Dupre, and A. Wylie. Oxford, UK: Oxford University Press.

Yli-Kuha, A. N., M. Gissler, R. Klemetti, R. Luoto, and E. Hemminki. 2012. Cancer morbidity in a cohort of 9175 Finnish women treated for infertility. *Human Reproduction* 27 (4):1149–55.

Zhao, Jing, Yanping Li, Qiong Zhang, and Yonggang Wang. 2015. Does ovarian stimulation for IVF increase gynaecological cancer risk? a systematic review and meta-analysis. *Reproductive Biomedicine Online* 31 (1):20–9.

Chapter 7

Different Things Delight Different People

On the Value-Neutrality of Reprogenetic Technologies

Introduction

Reprogenetic technologies, proponents contend, can provide human beings with an assortment of benefits. They serve to expand reproductive choices by allowing prospective parents to make decisions about the children they want to bring into existence (Harris 1998; Robertson 1994, 125; 2003; Savulescu 1999; Savulescu and Dahl 2000). At some point, supporters insist, these technologies will be used to create human beings who will live longer and healthier lives; enjoy better intellectual and artistic capacities such as verbal fluency, memory, spatial cognition, numerical ability, or musical talent; and generally achieve a greater degree of control over their own lives (Bostrom 2003; Buchanan 2011; Harris 2007; Savulescu 2005; Silver 1997). According to them, these increased capacities will ultimately benefit society by both reducing the burdens of disease and disability and creating people who can be more creative, productive, and morally sensitive.

Although usually at the behest of critics, reprogenetics advocates also recognize that these technologies can have negative impacts. For instance, sometimes they acknowledge that the use of reprogenetics might increase inequalities, result in overbearing parents, or contribute to discrimination against people thought to be disabled (DeGrazia 2012; Green 2007; Harris 2007; Savulescu 2005). Nonetheless, proponents argue that the reasonable answer to such risks is not interference with the development and implementation of these technologies but risk management via appropriate regulation.

The defense of reprogenetic technologies has thus been mostly limited to discussions about the risks and potential benefits of their use. Here, I challenge reprogenetic proponents' implicit or explicit assumption that an analysis of risks and benefits is all that is required when assessing the moral permissibility, or indeed the moral obligation, of using reprogenetic technologies. Underlying this assumption is a problematic conception of science and technology as value-neutral or value-free. In this chapter, I first discuss what such a conception involves. I then argue that this understanding of science and technology is inadequate for several reasons. First, it fails to acknowledge that values play an important role in science and technology in general, and thus it constitutes an implausible conceptualization of reprogenetics in particular. Second, it leads one to unjustifiably limit the ethical evaluation of reprogenetic technologies to an assessment of risks and benefits, usually very narrowly understood. Third, conceptions of science and technology as value-neutral render democratic participation in scientific and technological policy making superfluous or severely limited. Ultimately, I contend, the incorrect presupposition of value-neutrality impedes an ethically sound assessment of reprogenetic technologies. This chapter thus has two interrelated goals: to reject the value-neutrality thesis that underlies mainstream assessments of reprogenetics and to explore some of the ways in which these technologies are in fact value-laden.

That there is a close relationship between science and technology is uncontroversial. What that relationship consists in, however, is a matter of debate. Some conceptualize technology as applied science (Bunge 1966). According to this view, the aim of science is to provide us with empirically testable and true theories and laws that allow prediction of future events. Technology uses such theories and laws to intervene in and control reality so as to solve certain practical problems of concern to human beings. Other authors call attention to the ways in which technology actually makes possible new scientific knowledge (Pitt 2000). In this view, new instruments lead to the gathering of new data, which in turn leads to the development of new scientific theories. For others, science and technology represent a single complex rather than separate and distinguishable activities and practices (Bijker, Hughes, and Pinch 1987; Collins 1985; Latour 1987; MacKenzie and Wajcman 1985). This view of the relationship between science and technology underscores the similarity of their aims and emphasizes the importance of material artifacts in both. According to this account, experimentation, the basic staple of science, involves both the use of artifacts and interference with nature.[1]

I consider science and technology to be analytically distinct but closely connected social practices. It seems clear and uncontroversial that the development of reprogenetic technologies implicates both scientific and technological activities and knowledge and that they are intimately related. Knowledge about physiology, reproductive systems, and molecular biology is coupled with engineering capabilities and complex laboratory equipment

---

1. It is beyond the scope of this work to provide a review and evaluation of these different theoretical approaches (see, for instance, Cuevas 2005 and Radder 2009).

such as cooling devices, thermal cyclers, and microscopes, all of which also implicate knowledge of a variety of scientific disciplines. Although in what follows I discuss the value-neutrality thesis and its problems in relation to both science and technology, in general my claims about the value-laden nature of reprogenetic technologies will make no distinction between the role of values in the various scientific endeavors and the technological processes directly involved in reprogenetics.

The Value-Neutrality Thesis

One of the most persistent myths regarding science and technology is that these social practices are value-neutral. What exactly that means, however, is often vague. In this section, I seek to clarify what I take this thesis to entail. Let me begin with what I do not think this thesis mean. I do not interpret the value-neutrality thesis as defending the completely untenable claim that no values whatsoever play a role in scientific and technological research. Many who endorse this thesis recognize that epistemic or cognitive values play a necessary and central role in research (Betz 2013; Haack 1998; Mitchell 2004; Pitt 2000). Plausibly understood, then, the value-neutrality thesis refers only to contextual values, such as social, ethical, and political values. Further, I do not understand this thesis as denying any role whatsoever to contextual values. Indeed, many of those who defend the value-neutrality of science and technology accept that these values are relevant to a variety of decisions regarding these practices. For instance, it seems uncontroversial that contextual values are pertinent to decisions about whether and under what conditions human beings can be used as research subjects. In similar fashion, contextual values are accepted as important in considering what scientific and technological problems should be given priority in funding. That said, this role of values in science and technology is usually inappropriately considered irrelevant in the ethical assessment of science and technology.

In the case of the sciences, I take the value-neutrality thesis to amount to a denial that contextual values play any legitimate role in decisions concerning the gathering and characterization of evidence and the appraisal and acceptance of hypotheses (Haack 1998; Betz 2013; Mitchell 2004). In general, those who support the value-neutrality thesis see contextual values as detrimental to scientific knowledge. Indeed, it is not uncommon when rejecting the role of these values in science to use infamous cases that appear to demonstrate that whenever ethical, political, or other social values are brought into play, adverse consequences follow.

Proponents of the value-neutrality view argue that the history of science offers multiple examples supporting the claim that scientific research should be value-free. For instance, the well-known case of Russian horticulturist T. D. Lysenko, who directed work in Soviet agriculture toward methods and conclusions that supported a communist ideology, is often used as an illustration of the problems that result when contextual values are allowed to influence scientific research (Roll-Hansen 2005). Lysenko discarded scientific theories and frameworks in genetics and evolutionary biology not because they were empirically unsound but because he thought they were inconsistent with promoting collective farming and the specific political world view that underpinned Soviet agriculture. Be that as it may, it should be clear that the existence of instances—even multiple ones—in which use of contextual values led to bad science in no way constitutes evidence that such values *always* lead to disaster or that they *never* play legitimate roles in the production of scientific and technological knowledge. Likewise, accepting that contextual values play legitimate roles in science and technology does not commit one to accepting that such values are *always* appropriate or that they can *never* be unjustifiably used. Indeed, feminist scholars in science studies, who usually reject the value-neutrality thesis, have offered compelling evidence of the inappropriate use of contextual values (e.g., androcentric ones) in past and present scientific theories (e.g., Fausto-Sterling 1992; Lloyd 2005; Richardson 2012).

I also take the thesis that technologies are value-neutral to imply that technological developments are beneficial in general and instrumentally valuable in allowing us to attain goals with greater efficiency or to arrive at results that were previously unachievable. Technologies, from this perspective, can be put to good or bad use by human beings, but the technologies are themselves neutral instruments.[2] The often touted saying, "Guns don't kill people, people do," is a quintessential illustration of the value-neutrality thesis. Science and technology are thought to be mere tools for understanding and manipulating the world, with values entering in only when those tools are used (Pitt 2000). As should be clear, this view does not deny that technologies can have negative side effects. Part of the task of evaluating technological advances is indeed to assess the possibility of such negative impacts. But the value-neutral perspective attributes negative effects to faulty applications, immoral motivations, inadequate social policies, or a lack of sophistication in implementation: The problem is never with the technologies themselves. A hammer, it is often said by those who embrace the value-neutrality thesis, can be used to hang a portrait or to crack open a person's skull; guns can be used to kill innocent people or in just wars; nuclear power can be used to provide energy or to

---

2. Needless to say, rejecting the value-neutrality thesis does not commit one to denying that in some instances it might be appropriate to think of technologies as mere instruments that can be used appropriately or inappropriately. The rejection of this thesis involves a denial that the instrumental perspective is the only relevant one when reflecting on technologies.

build bombs; genetic technologies can be used to promote health or for racist purposes, but the hammer, gun, nuclear power, and genetics do not promote immoral use; they are merely tools.[3]

Proponents of reprogenetics arguably take these technologies to be value-free or value-neutral (Parens 2015). This is evidenced by their claims that it is the use or application of the technologies that may be a source for concern, rather than the technologies themselves. As Green contends:

> [T]he outcome of the debates probably depends on how well we implement the new technologies for choosing our genes. If we do so badly, gene modification will come under the shadow of the failed eugenic movement. If we implement it well, gene modification will become a routine and accepted part of our lives (Green 2007, 196).

Manifesting the value-neutrality thesis, advocates of reprogenetics remind us that although, as history clearly illustrates, genetic science and technology has been used for nefarious purposes, this does not mean that the technologies themselves embody immoral values (Agar 2005; Harris 2007; Savulescu and Kahane 2009; Robertson 2003). They recognize that genetic technologies and knowledge can be used to advance important and ethically appropriate human aims such as the promotion of health and the reduction of disease and its burdens. But they agree that in the wrong hands or under the wrong policies, these technologies can have negative impacts and be used to advance

3. Notice that the relevant question regarding the value-neutrality thesis is not about who is *causally* responsible for the bad effects of technologies. That is, rejecting the value-neutrality thesis need not involve rejecting the notion that causal responsibility for the bad effects rests with the users rather than with the technologies. The issue at stake is whether the negative impacts of technologies always and only result from some moral failing in the users—be those individuals or institutions.

immoral goals. In fact, advocates of reprogenetics note that this is what the Nazis did: They used genetic science and technology to exterminate thousands of human beings, to prevent people considered inferior from reproducing, and to strongly encourage those with desirable traits to procreate. Proponents believe that prospective parents today will use these technologies for appropriate goals, but they concede that prospective parents could decide to use reprogenetics, and physicians could help them, to have children with psychopathic or other undesirable characteristics. They claim, however, that there is nothing about the technologies themselves that necessitates such use. The problem is simply with the goals and motivations of the users of these technologies.

The value-neutrality thesis also underlies proponents' insistence that the immoral or potentially faulty applications of particular technologies are not an argument against the technologies themselves. For instance, when defending gene editing technologies, Harris and colleagues assert:

> It is true that GM [genetic modification] could be used for immoral purposes (for example, to produce biological weapons), but this is also true of any technology. It is also true that accidents with GM could lead to undesirable consequences (such as patient death through adverse reactions to particular gene therapy vectors). But the risk of accidental negative outcomes ought to be assessed and dealt with by a careful appraisal of the science involved.... However, concern over the possible negative consequences of GM cannot amount to a valid objection to DSA [deliberate sequence alteration] per se (Smith, Chan, and Harris 2012, 492).

Further evidence that proponents of reprogenetics take these technologies to be value-free is their insistence that regulation—rather than development of different kinds of technologies—is the way to deal with the potential negative consequences of their inappropriate use. As Savulescu and colleagues clearly state when defending, as a moral imperative, new gene editing technologies:

> IVF [in vitro fertilization] and PGD [preimplantation genetic diagnosis] can be used to select for traits like height and intelligence. This doesn't constitute a good reason not to use these technologies to avoid genetic disease. Rather than a blanket ban on research into gene editing technology, it would be more appropriate to ban the deployment of this technology to enhance normal traits, if that is the concern. Technology can and must be controlled by laws. And if it cannot, there is no point in making laws, including bans. Rather, energy would be better spent preparing to combat the unethical deployment of technology (Savulescu et al. 2015, 477).

Likewise, the exclusive attention that proponents give to narrowly understood risks and benefits of these technologies, and their explicit claims that these technologies are mere means to what advocates take to be ethically appropriate ends, constitute evidence that they take these technological innovations to be value-neutral. For instance, in his defense of enhancement technologies, Harris (2007) states:

> Our question is this: if the goal of enhanced intelligence, increased powers and capacities, and better health is something that we might strive to produce through education, including of course the more general health education of the community, why should we not produce these goals, if we can do so safely, through enhancement technologies or procedures? (2)

After all, Harris claims:

> [W]hat matters surely is the ethics of altering our nature, not the means that we adopt. If it's right to alter our nature, we should choose the best and most reliable, not to mention the most efficient and economical, methods of so doing (Harris 2007, 125).

Similarly, Savulescu takes different means to achieve the end of ensuring the well-being of our children as morally equivalent. In his words:

> Selective mating has been occurring in humans ever since time began. Facial asymmetry can reflect genetic disorder. Smell can tell us whether our mate will produce the child with the best resistance to disease. We compete for partners in elaborate mating games and rituals of display which sort the best matches from the worst. As products of evolution, we select our mates, both rationally and instinctively, on the basis of their genetic fitness—their ability to survive and reproduce. Our goal is the success of our offspring. With the tools of genetics, we can select offspring in a more reliable way (Savulescu 2005, 36).

What is Wrong with the Value-Neutrality Thesis?

Although belief in the value-neutrality of science and technology is common, it is questionable for a variety of reasons. It presents an implausible view of scientific and technological practices. Moreover, it has problematic implications for the evaluation of science and technology. Because contextual values are thought to be irrelevant, ethical analyses of reprogenetic technologies are limited to an assessment of risks and benefits, usually understood in narrow ways, which leads to neglect of other relevant normative concerns. Additionally, belief in the value-neutrality thesis renders democratic participation in decisions related to scientific and technological development and implementation unnecessary or very limited. In discussing these problems, I illustrate some of the ways in which reprogenetic technologies are value-laden. Of necessity, I will not seek to be exhaustive in this endeavor, so the discussion that follows should not be taken as giving an account of all that can be said about the value-laden nature of reprogenetics. Chapter 8, which addresses mitochondrial replacement techniques, will offer other illustrations of the interactions between reprogenetics and human societies.

Values in Science and Technology

A variety of studies have shown that the value-neutrality conception of science and technology is untenable. At a minimum, scientific and technological knowledge and development are goal-oriented processes. In general, a primary goal of science is not simply to discover truths about the world but to discover particularly *significant* truths. And such significance is determined by human values and interests (Duprè 1993; Kitcher 2001). Moreover, particular sciences, such as the biomedical sciences, have as an explicit social goal to improve human health. These social aims, and thus the values that underlie them, have implications that go beyond research priorities; they also help justify methodological choices. For instance, what the primary social aim of a particular medical intervention against human papilloma virus (HPV) infection is taken to be—whether to reduce cervical cancer morbidity and mortality, to reduce cervical cancer burdens in marginalized populations, or to produce a profitable drug—affects methodological decisions regarding the duration of clinical trials, the appropriate mix of subjects to be recruited, and the selection of biological endpoints (Intemann and de Melo-Martin 2010). Similarly, technological artifacts have specific functions: they are developed to do something or to be a component of a device that has some purpose. They can be used for particular goals but not for others, or at least not as effectively. Thus, even in a very minimal sense, the belief in the value-neutrality of reprogenetics is implausible.

Proponents of reprogenetics concede this minimal sense of value-ladenness and admit that scientific and technological knowledge is developed to serve some particular purpose or function. In the case of reprogenetic technologies, advocates take such purposes to be appropriate ones (e.g., improving human health, helping parents in their goal to ensure the well-being of their children, promoting human flourishing) even if they recognize that these technologies can be put to problematic uses.

But insisting that science and technology are not at all value-neutral involves more than recognizing that these practices have a goal or function. A substantial amount of scholarship has shown that scientific and technological knowledge is value-laden in more robust ways. Many have called attention to the legitimate role of contextual values in experimental design, choice of methodologies, characterization of the data, and interpretation of results. Contextual values might enter scientific decision-making through the use of background assumptions, for instance, because such assumptions are required to establish the relevance of empirical evidence to a hypothesis or a theory (Longino 1990). To illustrate, background assumptions, such as that there is a causal chain from genetic structures through anatomy to temperamental phenotypes, are needed to determine whether the increased presence of a particular allele in a given population will affect a particular phenotype such as shyness. In similar fashion, there are cases in which the content of scientific theories includes contextually normative concepts (Anderson 2004; Callicott, Crowder, and Mumford 1999; Dupré 2007; Elliott 2009). For example, research directed at measurement of harms to human health or the environment clearly involves normative concepts based on assumptions of what is central to well-being or the kinds of human or nonhuman interests that need protection (Anderson 2004; Shrader-Frechette 1991).

Even if the concepts in scientific theories might be thought to be merely descriptive, the choice of which conceptual frameworks to employ can be inextricably linked to contextual value judgments. For instance, in research on racial health disparities, the concept of "race" might be operationalized in a variety of apparently descriptive ways, such as the "one drop rule," the biological race of the mother, self-identification, or geographical ancestry. Ultimately, though, the decision of how to classify races depends on contextual value judgments about what one takes to be salient about racial health disparities (de Melo-Martin and Intemann 2007). Moreover, acceptance or rejection of hypotheses usually happens in the context of uncertainty. Hence, scientists must consider whether there is enough evidence to accept or reject a particular hypothesis or interpretation of the evidence. This involves considering not only the likelihood of error but also how bad the consequences would be should one be wrong. Scientists thus need to make ethical value judgments about which sorts of errors are acceptable and which are not (Douglas 2009; Rudner 1953; Shrader-Frechette 1991).

Scholars in science and technology studies and in philosophy of technology have also shown that the relationship between contextual values and technological development and implementation is significantly more intimate than what proponents of reprogenetics acknowledge. Values affect the decisions that various stakeholders, including engineers, make when developing particular technologies (van de Poel 2001). Some researchers have also called attention to the ways in which technologies can exhibit political qualities (Feenberg 1999; Habermas 1971; Winner 1980, 1986). In some cases, the design, invention, or implementation of a technology can support or exclude particular political values. For instance, an artifact as apparently innocuous as a bridge can be intentionally designed with an overhead clearance too low to allow bus traffic, reserving its use to cars (Winner 1980). In a context in which only poor people and racial and ethnic minorities use public transportation, such a bridge would have the intentional effect of limiting access to certain people. But technologies can embody specific forms of power and authority even when there has been no intentionality on the part of the designers (Winner 1986). For example, because of the highly dangerous weaponry that can result from byproducts of nuclear power, its use requires a centralized, rigid, and hierarchical social structure. Solar energy, on the other hand, is more compatible with a decentralized and non-hierarchical social system.

Technologies also influence our perception of the world and our behavior; they mediate human actions (Borgmann 1984; Ihde 1990; Latour 1993; Verbeek 2005). They disclose reality in new ways and shape our perceptions of the world and of the entities that inhabit it. Think, for instance, of telescopes and microscopes and the ways in which these technologies have shaped how we perceive and conceptualize reality (Idhe 1993). Or consider the ways in which prenatal ultrasound technology influences perceptions of the fetus (Duden 1993; Verbeek 2008). It constitutes the fetus as a separate entity and the pregnant woman as the "environment'" within which the fetus develops; it also transforms the fetus into a patient, one who can be diagnosed with certain conditions (Chervenak and McCullough 1996). X-rays, magnetic resonance imaging (MRI) scans, and sonograms allow clinicians access to the interior of our bodies. Microscopes disclose a realm of microorganisms completely inaccessible to the naked eye. Space telescopes help us reach beyond the confines of our own galaxy.

Reprogenetic technologies similarly inform people's perceptions and behaviors. They interact with social, ethical, and political values to shape reality in epistemically and morally relevant ways. One such aspect of reality that has been influenced by reprogenetic technologies is the embryo. Embryos, like fetuses, are contested entities: This is evinced in the attention paid by critics and proponents of reprogenetics to their moral status. Before the advent of IVF, concerns about the moral status of extracorporeal embryos would have been of little importance. The moral status of the embryo only moved to center stage when these reprogenetic technologies made possible the creation of embryos outside a woman's body. Moreover, these technologies brought about the reconfiguration of the embryo: Where once we just had embryos, we now have "spared embryos," "pre-embryos," "fertilized eggs," and so on (Maienschein 2002).

Furthermore, reprogenetic technologies, as we have seen, aim not simply at helping infertile people to have genetically related offspring. Their goals go further, providing prospective parents with a better chance of having a "healthier" child, a "better" child, or an "enhanced" child. The availability of these technologies thus shape our understanding of embryos in other ways. First, embryos are conceptualized as "healthy" or ' "unhealthy," of good or bad "quality," depending on whether they have or lack specific characteristics desired by prospective parents.[4] Second, they are constituted as "patients" who can be diagnosed with particular diseases or disabilities and whose suffering can apparently be prevented. And, with the use of enhancement techniques, they can be "treated," "bettered," or "enhanced."

---

4. Or by scientists, if the embryos are used only for research purposes.

Another aspect of reality shaped by reprogenetic technologies is the understanding of health and disease—indeed, the understanding of well-being itself. Health, disease, disability, and well-being are thought of as pertaining to, and are often reduced to, molecular aspects of human biology. Because they offer the capability of assessing the embryo's genome, these technologies seem to allow us to predict whether a future child will be deaf, disabled, healthy, intelligent, a boy or a girl and whether the child will have musical talent, self-control, a sense of humor, a sunny temperament, and so on. Of course, the emphasis on molecular genetics when conceptualizing human traits and behaviors in general, and health and disease in particular, is hardly new (Lewontin, Rose, and Kamin 1984; Lippman 1992; Nelkin and Lindee 1995; Oyama 1985; Tabery 2014). Genes and genomes are given a privileged causal status in our explanations of multiple human traits, including, but not limited to, those related to health and disease. Even when other factors, such as other biological or environmental aspects, are considered to be playing a causal role, genetic factors are thought to be causative in a way that is fundamentally different from all the other material factors known to be involved. But this is precisely the consequence of the value-laden nature of science and technology: Reprogenetic technologies are shaped by the privileging of genetic causes, and at the same time, the use of these technologies reinforces this privileging. Indeed, as we saw in Chapter 5, in spite of the fact that everyone ostensibly agrees that "nature" and "nurture" interact in complex ways, current use of reprogenetics is hard to understand without presupposing genetic determinism. Recall that the aim of these technologies is to select particular kinds of embryos by virtue of the fact that they have or lack certain genetic mutations or variants. Similarly, the purported goal of enhancement technologies is to manipulate the human genome under the assumption that such manipulations will produce a desired phenotypic trait.

Technologies also mediate our practical options and, with them, the reasons we have to act (Latour 2005; Verbeek 2005; Waelbers 2011). They allow us to do some things, expanding some options, constraining others, and altering still others. Speed bumps, for instance, force us to slow down (Latour 1994). The introduction of e-mail has increased our options to stay in touch with family and friends but has also transformed not just the speed but the content of our communications. Or consider, again, ultrasound and similar prenatal technologies, which have transformed the experience of pregnancy by, for example, presenting prospective parents, and particularly women, with choices they did not have before, such as choosing whether or not to have an abortion because the fetus has been diagnosed with some health problem (Rothman 1987).

The transforming nature of technology is also evident in reprogenetic technologies. Insofar as these technologies shape reality, they influence our responses to it. For instance, in conceptualizing embryos as healthy or unhealthy "patients" whose suffering can be prevented through use of these technologies, it appears that prospective parents' choices can contribute to a reduction of disease, disability, or decreased well-being. But this is done not by curing the "patient" but by ensuring that a particular child is not born. Whatever suffering might have occurred is prevented by precluding existence. Whether or not one thinks that this is a difference of moral import, it is one masked by reprogenetic technologies' constitution of embryos as patients.

Constructing embryos as patients also calls for new means to attend to the needs of these "patients." With these technologies, clinicians can *diagnose* particular genetic mutations implicated in diseases and disabilities. Unsurprisingly, this seems to call for the development and implementation of technological practices to help *treat* such diseases and disabilities. As might be expected, then, gene editing technologies appear as the most appropriate of responses from this perspective. Just like any other patient, embryos could be *cured* or *fixed* and their well-being ensured with the help of these new technologies.

Similarly, the construction of health, disease, and well-being as pertaining to the genome also calls for particular kinds of responses. If disease, disability, and other conditions that can contribute to well-being are primarily encountered at the genetic level, then reprogenetic technologies appear as an efficient solution to those concerns. Thus, without denying that other organismal and environmental factors are relevant, the diagnostic capacities of new technologies constitute a powerful case for intervening at the genomic level.

Moreover, reprogenetic technologies transform these aspects of the human condition into primarily individual problems. Attending to the well-being of one's children, to their health and their abilities, becomes the exclusive responsibility of prospective parents, and particularly of women. Prospective parents are in charge of managing risks to health and quality of life. They have the task of fulfilling the promises of reprogenetic technologies: minimizing the existence of diseases, disorders, and disabilities; increasing the welfare of their children; and outperforming evolution by choosing specific traits, as Harris (2007) would have it. Reprogenetic technologies thus contribute to a more and more widespread reliance on individuals to manage their own health risks and the risks to well-being (Clarke 2010; Conrad 2007; Foucault 2008; Rose 2007).

Reprogenetic technologies reinforce the individualization of what are, to a significant extent, collective problems and embody, in and of themselves, such individualization. Thanks to reprogenetic technologies, a variety of human traits appear amenable to intervention, including diseases such as Tay Sachs, Huntington's, or cancer; mental health problems such as anxiety, attention deficit hyperactivity disorder, neuroticism, or schizophrenia;

impairments such as deafness or blindness; and conditions such as alcoholism, criminal behavior, and substance addiction. Also open to intervention are traits that affect human character and temperament, such as aggression, optimism, sense of humor, shyness, sympathy, novelty seeking, altruism, and, of course, assorted cognitive capacities such as intelligence and memory. Even sexual preference is included as a trait open to "treatment" (Savulescu 2001, 417).

All of these traits are biomedicalized, consigned to the realm of individual choice rather than the territory of collective solutions. Individuals are classified as "at risk" of passing on to their offspring particular genetic traits that can affect their children's welfare. Individuals are therefore called to manage their responsibility and encouraged—sometimes even morally required—to make use of technological advances that presumably allow them to reduce or eliminate such risks. In fact, these technologies, particularly those directed at enhancing human traits, transform all prospective parents into individuals "at risk." After all, enhancement techniques would allow all of them to "improve" the genetic endowment of their embryos in multiple ways. But although the "at risk" category has been massively extended, managing these risks is still deemed an individual responsibility. Management consists in either ensuring that embryos with particular characteristics are not brought into existence or, insofar as our technical abilities will ever be able to accomplish it, manipulating embryos' genetic endowment so as to enhance desired traits.

In addition to influencing our perceptions of what is real, the problems encountered, and our responses to those problems, technologies can also alter and shape our moral beliefs (Swierstra and Waelbers 2012). Of course, insofar as technological innovations influence our perceptions of reality and of the realm of possibility, they also have consequences for the morality of our actions. For example, construction of the embryo as a patient calls for specific moral responses (i.e., treatment). But technologies also affect morality itself. Indeed, one of the most obvious ways in which technologies are value-laden is that they affect our ideas of what is right or wrong, virtuous or vicious, good or bad, morally obligatory or forbidden. Their influence on such questions can result from their transformative impact on what is valued or the extent to which something is valued. For instance, our understanding of the good of friendship is arguably being transformed by the use of social networking (Froding and Peterson 2012; Vallor 2012). New technological innovations can also create new moral duties. For example, our ability to harvest organs has created a moral duty to become organ donors. Genetic technologies present people with moral questions about whether to acquire genetic information about themselves and others in order to make appropriately informed decisions (Rhodes 1998).

Technologies can also reinforce particular norms, at least in part because such norms are inscribed in the technologies in both clear and subtle ways. IVF, for example, has undoubtedly served to buttress gender norms about responsibility for reproduction. Similarly, although more subtly and contested, reproductive technologies have also contributed to reinforcing kinship bio-genetic norms (Zeiler and Malmquist 2014; Birenbaum-Carmeli 2009; Haslanger 2009; Crabb and Augoustinos, 2008). Likewise, the normative judgments we use to evaluate new technologies co-evolve with the introduction of those technologies (Jasanoff 2004). Some of those changes are subtle and may go unnoticed, whereas others are revolutionary. Changes in sexual mores, for instance, cannot be disconnected from the introduction of the pill. Interestingly, this phenomenon is actually often used as an argument against criticisms of new technologies. It is not unusual for their proponents to remind critics that technologies such as blood transfusion, anesthesia, and IVF were once fervently rejected and thought to threaten the moral order but have now been embraced by society to such an extent that it is deemed unethical to prevent people from having access to them.

Reprogenetic technologies also influence our values, moral norms, and moral beliefs. One of the obvious ways in which they do so is by generating new moral obligations and shaping the ways in which particular moral obligations are conceptualized. This goes beyond the fact that the introduction of new technologies can give rise to internal or external pressures promoting their use—although, as we saw in earlier chapters, reprogenetic technologies certainly have this effect. They can also transform the ways in which moral demands are conceptualized. For example, there is little doubt that prospective parents have a pro tanto moral obligation to attend to the well-being of their future children. What that obligation entails depends, of course, on a variety of factors. If reprogenetic technologies are available, such an obligation is constituted in a very particular fashion, as the moral obligation to ensure that embryos with particular kinds of traits thought to decrease well-being are not brought into existence. Indeed, as discussed in Chapter 4, this view is explicitly defended by proponents of reprogenetics. The moral obligation to attend to the well-being of our children is transformed into the moral obligation to select the best child one can have and the obligation to enhance one's offspring.

The fact that reprogenetic technologies now present the option of having a *chosen* child calls attention to yet another way in which these technologies transform ethical values. By introducing the possibility of choosing among embryos, these technologies alter current normative conceptions of parenting. Not that common normative notions of parenting are inconsistent with prospective parents' making any choices at all. Clearly, our ordinary understanding of what makes a good parent is compatible with choosing *when* to have a child or *how many* children to have. And indeed, a variety of technological innovations, from contraceptive methods to reproductive technologies, now allow prospective parents to make just such choices and to do so in more efficient ways. But choosing one's children challenges a widely accepted, and arguably appropriate, normative notion of parenting, one that calls for parents to love whatever child comes along (Herissone-Kelly 2007, 2007; McDougall 2005; Scully, Shakespeare, and Banks 2006). Such a challenge is most obvious when the traits chosen are thought to be trivial characteristics that have nothing to do with the well-being of the future child. As we have seen, reprogenetic technologies today allow the selection of some such characteristics, such as sex, a trait that proponents of reprogenetics explicitly acknowledge is morally neutral. Advocates believe that in the future similarly trivial traits, such as hair color or perfect pitch, might also be available for selection.

Notice that this is not an argument that reprogenetic technologies will make parents more critical of their children if they ultimately do not express the traits for which their parents were attempting to select, or that parents will love their children less. It might well be the case that parents end up loving their children even if they are not what they wished for (Green 2007).[5] Rather, the effects that reprogenetic technologies have on normative conceptions of parenting illustrate their value-laden nature. That parents will still love their children is beside the point and in no way makes the effects of these technologies on parenting notions any less real. After all, it is one thing to be loved in spite of one's

5. Whether this will or will not be the case is in large part an empirical question. Proponents of reprogenetics seem quite confident that parents will uncondition-ally love their children even if the latter fail to have the characteristics chosen for them. I am somewhat less sanguine about this possibility. After all, if prospective parents go through the expensive, time-consuming, risky (for women), and stress-ful task of choosing a particular child, it is not unreasonable to believe that they might be more than a little disappointed if the child in question is not what they expected.

characteristics, and quite another to be loved irrespective of such characteristics. Reprogenetic technologies are thus challenging widely accepted normative conceptions of parenting.

Of course, that science and technology are not value-neutral but value-laden in a variety of ways is not an argument against science and technology. Indeed, as many have argued, not only is it false to contend that contextual value judgments undermine the objectivity or rationality of science, but their use can actually result in better science and technology (Anderson 2004; Dupré 2007; Harding 1998; Longino 2002). However, recognizing that science and technology are indeed value-laden calls for reflection upon those values, for critical evaluation of how they affect and are affected by scientific and technological innovations, and for taking such effects into account when deciding what technologies to develop and implement.

The Need for More Than Risks and Benefits

The value-neutrality thesis is inadequate not simply because it fails to offer an accurate view of scientific and technological knowledge and practices. It also severely limits the ethical assessment of scientific and technological developments. Such an approach places the production of scientific and technological knowledge in one sphere and the use of such knowledge via practical applications in a completely different one: Scientists and engineers produce knowledge and develop artifacts; users put the knowledge and devices to work. Ethical questions are raised only at the application stage, and they usually concern the moral responsibilities of users. Humanists and social scientists are charged with evaluating the ethical and social implications of scientific and technological knowledge and devices. They are tasked with assessing their risks and potential benefits of use.

As indicated earlier, this is exactly what the debate about reprogenetics has focused on. Advocates dedicate their time to presenting us with an array of actual, possible, and imagined benefits that individuals and society can derive from the use of reprogenetic technologies. Some such benefits were mentioned earlier and include the possibilities that our offspring will have longer lives, be free from severe diseases and disabilities, and be able to enjoy life more fully (DeGrazia 2012; Harris 2007, 2015; Savulescu 2005, 2006; Savulescu et al. 2015; Silver 1997; Smith, Chan, and Harris 2012). Reprogenetic technologies, proponents contend, can also help ensure that our children are more intelligent and better able to deal with their environments. Similarly, advocates hold that enhancement technologies could be directed to improving traits that are constitutive of autonomy, such as our concept of self, the capacity to form and act on conceptions of the good life, and the ability to predict and pay attention to the consequences of behavior (Savulescu 2006). They could also be aimed at improving our offspring's moral character and thus used to produce people who are more loving, sympathetic, compassionate, or just and who have better motives (Savulescu and Persson 2012). Supporters argue that all of these improvements will provide benefits, not only to those who have been selected or enhanced but also to society in general, because ultimately they are likely to result in increased productivity and more just societies (Buchanan 2008). In fact, the presumed benefits of reprogenetic technologies are so expansive that when reading the works of proponents it is difficult to avoid the impression that these technologies constitute the solution to all of the problems humanity faces. Gene editing technologies are said to have enormous therapeutic potential:

> Roughly 6% of all births have a serious birth defect, which is genetic or partly genetic in origin. . . . Advanced and precise gene editing techniques could virtually eradicate genetic

birth defects, thereby benefiting nearly 8 million children every year. In addition 35% of all deaths are due to chronic diseases, such as cancer and diabetes, in those under 70. Gene editing could significantly lower this disease burden thereby benefiting billions of people around the world over time (Savulescu et al. 2015, 476).

In the case of mitochondrial replacement interventions, we are asked to celebrate:

the advent of a new and life-enhancing therapy and the impressive science that enables this generation, and future ones, to correct the mistakes inherent in so-called normal sexual reproduction and to continue to lighten, where we can, the burden of human existence (Harris 2015, 11).

The survival of humanity itself is said to be at stake. The existence of wars, famines, inequality, severe poverty, and global warming makes it such an urgent matter

to improve humanity morally to the point that it can responsibly handle the powerful resources of modern technology that we should seek whatever means there are to effect this. If, contrary to what we believe, we could achieve this moral improvement by cognitive means, all well and good. But if it takes moral bioenhancement, these should also be sought and applied, alongside the cognitive means. The future of life on Earth might well hinge upon the adoption of this policy (Persson and Savulescu 2013, 130).

Given the enormous potential benefits that these technologies are said to bring, it is unsurprising that proponents are not particularly impressed with the risks. Indeed, they claim that we should be wary of preventing the development of these technologies because of what they take to be conjectures about serious risks to individuals or to society. As Savulescu and colleagues insist in the case of gene editing techniques:

> There are clear moral reasons to continue with gene editing research. Advanced gene editing techniques could reduce the global burden of genetic disease and potentially benefit millions worldwide. This research is a moral imperative. It does indeed raise profound ethical issues but these are best addressed with ethical debate and judicious, selective legislation to prevent abuse and premature use of this promising technology (Savulescu et al. 2015, 478).

Of course, proponents of reprogenetics also consider the risks of these technologies, albeit grudgingly. But their risk considerations tend to be quite limited. Although in general advocates do not address them in any significant way, risks to health are obviously thought relevant. For the most part, proponents simply acknowledge that the use of these technologies is predicated on their being safe, or safe enough, and effective. Undeniably, during the research stage, there will be uncertainty about the safety of these procedures, but advocates contend that this is the case for all interventions. For them, so long as appropriate preclinical studies exist to show that the technologies are reasonably safe and effective and women and their partners are appropriately informed about risks and uncertainties, then proceeding with clinical research in reprogenetics does not raise unusual moral concerns.

The attention proponents give to other types of risks usually depends on the kinds of objections they are attempting to address. Their discussions tend to be directed toward either dismissing critics' concerns about most risks or offering assurances that such risks can be appropriately managed. For instance, critics have argued that some parents, having spent considerable amount of time and presumably money in selecting and enhancing their offspring, might come to see their children as mere products of their wills (Kass 2002). They might also become overbearing, disillusioned, and unloving if their children do not live up to their expectations. Advocates often dismiss these worries by indicating that the existence of overbearing parents does not depend on the use of reprogenetics. Furthermore, they claim that rather than creating overbearing and disappointed parents, the use of reprogenetic technologies is likely to result in more loving and dedicated ones, partly because some parents might find it easier to care for and love a child who is brighter, more beautiful, and healthier than she would have been without the use of reprogenetics (Green 2007; Robertson 2003). They also tend to be dismissive of concerns by critics that these technologies might contribute to discrimination against people with disabilities (Asch 1999, 2003; Parens and Asch 1999; Scully 2008; Stangl 2010), contending that such fears are overstated (Harris 2001, 2005). For advocates, the fact that prospective parents use reprogenetic technologies to have children free of disabilities is in no way an instance of discrimination against disabled people or an indication that people with disabilities are not equal and should not be treated as such (Buchanan et al. 2000; DeGrazia 2012; Harris 2001; Savulescu and Kahane 2009). Some proponents of reprogenetics also argue that these technologies will likely result in a decreased incidence of some disabilities and this could lead to more assistance for those who are still affected, so that they would be more likely to live full lives with the help of a variety of technological and social supports (Bostrom 2003).

But if one rejects the assumption that science and technology are value-neutral, then limiting ethical evaluations to the often narrowly understood risks and benefits of use will be inadequate. Assessment of the risks and potential benefits of the development and implementation of particular technological advances is certainly a necessary aspect of any ethical evaluation, but it is hardly sufficient. If values are an inextricable aspect of science and technology, a variety of normative concerns will be germane to the ethical assessment of particular technologies. First, considerations about the ways in which problems are constituted or framed are surely important. When the framing of a problem is neglected, we fail to perceive how such framing influences the perceived validity of solutions. In the case of reprogenetic technologies, the focus on risks and potential benefits of using these technologies leads us to ignore the fact that the problem is framed as a narrow inquiry into the best way to use them to improve human well-being safely and efficiently. If the problem is framed as determining how biomedical technologies can be used to improve health or increase human intelligence, strength, or life span, the appropriate solutions will be very different from those proposed if the problem is framed as, for example, trying to determine the various ways in which such improvements can be achieved. In the first case, the most significant concerns will be related to technological improvements, but in the second case, social and political responses will also be of relevance.

Second, equally as significant as any ethically sound evaluation of new technological developments are upstream questions about the work of scientists and engineers, their assumptions, the values underlying their projects, the utility of such programs, and the values embodied by new technologies. So also are questions about how the practices and values of knowledge production influence the types of technologies that are developed and how these practices and values affect those technologies that are found to be desirable or even feasible. For instance, the focus on molecular factors as causal mechanisms in health and disease makes the use of genetic technologies as diagnostic tools important in our desire to reduce disease burdens. At the same time, as I discussed earlier, the existence of these technologies reinforces the role of molecular genetics in scientific explanations of health and disease.

Third, the focus on narrowly conceived risks and potential benefits that follows from the conceptualization of science and technology as value-neutral also wrongly precludes reflection on the value of specific goals (de Melo-Martin 2010). As mentioned, proponents of reprogenetic technologies take the goals that these technologies will presumably help us to achieve as uncontroversially desirable: increasing reproductive choices, reducing the burdens of disease and disability, and improving human flourishing.[6] Nonetheless, although one might value these goals, it might still be quite appropriate to consider whether they should be pursued. A variety of equally valuable goals often co-exist in a context in which the time and resources available are limited. If so, a critical evaluation of the goals that we seek to attain is necessary to allow appropriate decisions about which goals to pursue and when. An appropriate assessment of reprogenetics ought not to sidestep such questions.

It is also important to evaluate the ways in which goals are characterized. Consider the goal of promoting human flourishing that reprogenetic technologies will supposedly help us achieve. Most people would likely endorse human flourishing as a desirable goal, but what human flourishing involves is certainly a matter of debate. Is increased intelligence or physical strength constitutive of human flourishing? Is musical talent or possessing a particular hair color? Likewise, even if many would agree that reducing disabilities is a worthy aim, there is considerable

---

6. And, if the claims of many proponents of reprogenetics are to be believed, saving the planet and the human species.

disagreement about what constitutes disability and whether all disabilities should be targeted or only specific ones (Davis 2013; Watson, Roulstone, and Thomas 2012). If some should be targeted, to what extent? "Human flourishing" is a banner term that encourages support while distracting attention from what exactly marches under its cover. Therefore, a critical assessment of what is entailed by the pursuit of espoused goals should not be ignored.

Fourth, the understanding of science and technology as value-neutral and the focus on risks and benefits stand in the way of careful consideration of the relationship between means and ends and the appropriateness of specific means. As I indicated earlier, in the debate over reprogenetics, proponents are quick to argue that differences between means are of little ethical importance (Buchanan 2011; Harris 2007; Savulescu 2005). For them, only the goal is relevant: If reprogenetic technologies can help us achieve that goal in more efficient ways, nothing else matters. Of course, this presupposes that the means in question—reprogenetic technologies—are indeed appropriate to achieve those goals. But this is a very big assumption indeed. Clearly, even if we were to grant that reprogenetic technologies can reduce disease and disability, the fact that they can do so is not, by itself, sufficient to support the development and implementation of these technologies. Doubtless, there are many means of attaining this specific aim that most people would be unwilling to deem appropriate, even if they are highly effective. If reprogenetic technologies are thought to constitute appropriate means to achieve some desirable goals, it seems clear that considering whether they are the best means and not just the most efficient ones, or whether alternative means would be more suitable, is an essential component of a sound ethical assessment of any technological advance. Hence, even if one were to agree that particular risks and potential benefits are likely to result from the development and use of reprogenetic technologies, and even if one were to concur that the balance of risks and benefits is a reasonable one, one could still legitimately ask whether reprogenetic technologies are a suitable way to respond to peoples' desire to promote their children's well-being or whether other means would be more ethically suitable.

Fifth, concerns about uncertainties—both what we know is unknown and what we do not even suspect—are clearly important to any adequate technology assessment (Jonas 1984; Wynne 2001). Although technical risk-benefit calculations do consider uncertainties, the focus on risks and potential benefits in the ethical analysis of these technologies usually obscures concerns about uncertainties in knowledge and conceals the limits of even the best scientific data. The language of risks reduces issues of uncertainty, ambiguity, and ignorance to the more controllable and deterministic processes usually associated with risks analysis. This is important, and not only because serious harms might result that had not been predicted at all. Attention to uncertainties in ethical evaluations of reprogenetics is also imperative because it allows for a more careful consideration regarding which strategies (both institutional and individual) should be developed to best deal with such unknown consequences. Significant uncertainties, known and unknown, exist concerning some of the newest reprogenetic technologies, such as gene editing and mitochondrial replacement. The qualitative differences between those and other reproductive or genetic technologies are such that careful attention is required to ensure that relevant aspects are not ignored, constructed as unknowable, or thought to be already known (Proctor and Schiebinger 2008). For instance, focusing on some of the risks to women's health that result from the use of reprogenetics, such as ovarian hyperstimulation or multiple pregnancies, obscures much that is unknown about the health effects of the drugs used and particularly about the long-term effects of these drugs and procedures on women and children. Because these uncertainties are usually neglected, researchers simply fail to study such effects, ensuring that the uncertainties continue to prevail. As I said in chapter 1, the need to attend to uncertainties is not an irrational demand for complete knowledge but a call to recognize that there is more to analyzing technologies in ethically appropriate ways than simply assessing known risks and potential benefits. Finally, insofar as technologies embody particular values, shape and transform others, change the ways we perceive and interact with reality, and affect the kinds of solutions that are thought possible, a sound evaluation of scientific and technological developments surely requires attention to these effects. Consider, for example, my contention that reprogenetic technologies present problems about health, disease, and well-being as individuals' medical problems. Focusing exclusively on risks and benefits as typically conceptualized fails to attend to the consequences of individualizing these problems. Individualization both removes concerns about health and quality of life from the social context in which they are relevant and neglects the prospect of collective solutions. The simple fact that most of the traits that these technologies set out to manipulate affect an individual's quality of life in one way or another does not in and of itself make these problems primarily individual ones. Not only can issues about health, disease, disability, well-being, and quality of life be addressed in collective fashion; arguably, doing so should often be the primary response. After all, whether many of these traits constitute a disadvantage or negatively affect one's quality of life depends very much on the social context in which they are expressed. In a society where access to gluten-free products is common, for example, having an intolerance to gluten would not constitute much of a problem. Likewise, societies that are completely accepting of homosexuality would undermine any attempt to justify selecting against such a trait on the grounds that it affected people's quality of life.

Moreover, even for traits that arguably would negatively affect people's well-being in any human society, minimizing or disregarding the relevance of collective solutions is problematic. It is well known that conditions of material deprivation, such as inadequate nutrition and lack of access to appropriate housing or to clean water and sanitation, constitute health risks and increase mortality (CSDH 2008; Daniels 2008; Marmot et al. 2012). Even if absolute deprivation is not an issue, a variety of social determinants such as income, education, occupational rank, social class, and social support greatly affect people's health and quality of life. What societies we have, how they are structured, what resources are available to people, and how resources are distributed are all factors that significantly influence people's health and well-being. Collective actions, and not simply individual ones mediated by biomedicine, are needed to address concerns related to these social determinants.

Given the relevance of collective approaches to improving health and well-being, assessments of reprogenetic technologies that obscure or ignore their impact on society at large are clearly inadequate. Such assessments will inevitably fail to attend to the fact that, whatever degree of control these technologies afford prospective parents in trying to improve the health and quality of life of their future children, the focus on individual solutions unjustifiably overburdens them. In a social context in which women are thought to be particularly responsible for the well-being of children, the emphasis on individual solutions is likely to contribute to the already intense scrutiny of women's reproductive decisions.

Such assessments will also fail to reflect on the ways in which the individualization and privatization of concerns about health and quality of life shifts the responsibility to individuals and is thus likely to negatively affect collective efforts. Insofar as prospective parents are charged with ensuring that their children have the types of physical, psychological, and cognitive traits thought to improve well-being, policies that ignore the social determinants of health and well-being are likely to flourish. Such an approach could inappropriately divert attention and resources away from the social, political, and economic factors that have such a significant impact on health, disease, and well-being. Given that genetic factors are only one of many complex elements affecting quality of life, neglecting the social determinants of health will only serve to worsen people's health and quality of life.

Likewise, if, as I have argued, reprogenetic technologies challenge widely accepted normative notions of parenting, an appropriate assessment needs to take this into account. The desirability of such a transformation should be addressed, as well as its effects on the relationships between children and their parents. Given the relevance of families for societies in general (Brighouse and Swift 2014), such considerations are of no small matter and should be included in any analysis of reprogenetic technologies. Similarly, if reprogenetic technologies incorporate values about what constitutes desirable and undesirable human lives, as they clearly do, then these values ought to be critically evaluated. A sound, robust ethical assessment would also require reflection upon the ways in which new technological developments influence or transform individual choices and preferences, which moral aspects they make salient, which ones they obscure, and how they shape reality.

How much importance should be given to these considerations when ethically assessing reprogenetic technologies is obviously a matter of debate. That they are important is, I believe, indisputable. Conceptualizing science and technology as value-neutral and emphasizing the evaluation of narrowly conceived risks and benefits simply conceals the moral relevance of these concerns and thus impedes a robust and sound ethical evaluation of these technologies.

Democratic Participation

A further problem with a conception of science and technology as value-neutral is that it severely restricts or renders pointless democratic participation in scientific and technological development (Habermas 1971; Irwin and Wynne 1996; Jasanoff 1990; Shrader-Frechette 1991). If science and technology are thought to be value-neutral, then the only relevant factors in the evaluation of knowledge production and technological innovations would be scientific and technical issues. Given that only scientists and engineers have the necessary scientific and technical expertise, their opinions alone would be pertinent for assessing a technology. The value-neutrality thesis makes critical analysis and input from citizens at various stages of decision making not just unnecessary but inappropriate, given that citizens in general fail to have sufficient relevant knowledge. Their participation could only serve to delay or, worse, impede scientific and technological progress.

This does not mean that those endorsing the value-neutrality thesis deem democratic decisions regarding all aspects of science and technology superfluous. Clearly, as I mentioned earlier, even if one accepts that science and technology are value-neutral, one can still concede that citizens should have some say about whether to fund particular types of scientific and technological developments and about whether, and if so how, to regulate others. For instance, governments can ban the use of certain pesticides if they are found to be dangerous to people's health or can regulate the use of X-ray devices to reduce unnecessary radiation exposure. Citizen-wide discussion about what goals to pursue would seem consistent with the value-neutrality thesis, but once the goals are agreed upon, debate about scientific and technological developments would be reduced to questions about safety and efficacy. Similarly, democratic participation at the application stage can also be made to fit the conceptualization of science and technology as value-neutral. Although, as we have seen, proponents of reprogenetics usually dismiss most arguments about risks related to these technologies, they agree that insofar as some risks result from their use, regulations are appropriate. Recall, for instance, the use of reprogenetic technologies for sex selection for social reasons. Even though proponents of reprogenetics tend to argue that serious risks or harms are unlikely to follow from this practice, they concede that if the use of sex selection resulted in a severe sex ratio imbalance, it would be appropriate to regulate it (Harris 2007; Robertson 2003; Savulescu 1999). Democratic participation in these cases would also be consistent with the value-neutrality thesis.

However, if scientific and technological knowledge is value-laden, democratic participation cannot be limited to the application of technological developments. Insofar as technologies are not mere instruments, many other decisions should be open to democratic input rather than left only to experts. Clearly, questions about how to conceptualize particular goals are hardly the kinds of decisions that should be left in the hands of scientific and technological experts. These professionals might be best placed to determine whether particular technological solutions will be good or efficient means to achieve a certain end, but they have neither the relevant expertise nor the legitimate authority to decide how to understand the end in question. Moreover, even if one were to concede that technology assessment necessitates only the evaluation of risks and potential benefits narrowly understood, this hardly legitimates expert decision making.

Determination and analysis of risks, harms, and benefits is not, in and of itself, a value-neutral activity (Douglas and Wildavsky 1982; Shrader-Frechette 1991). As we saw in Chapter 3, determination of what counts as a harm or a risk presupposes a host of normative considerations. Events do not come labeled as "I am a risk" or "I am a benefit"; on the contrary, such determinations involve value judgments about what matters to human beings. Considerations about how risky is too risky (or not risky enough), how compelling benefits are, what the relevant time frame for investigating risks is, the extent to which risks proposed are manageable, and what standards are to be used to determine the absence of unmanageable risks are all value-laden judgments.

Furthermore, even if one assumes that the magnitude, probability, and significance of the risks are acceptable and that the balance of risks and benefits of using reprogenetic technologies falls squarely on the side of the benefits, an appropriate risk assessment must also consider whether other alternatives exist that might prove less risky or offer greater benefits; this also requires value judgments. Similarly, when trying to balance risks and potential benefits, one must also make judgments about how much greater benefits have to be to outweigh associated risks. Recall for instance, the different value judgments that play a role in determining whether sex selection practices promote sexism—judgments about what constitutes sexism, what to count as evidence for sexism, how serious the potential harm could be, and so on. Likewise, determining, say, whether the risk of parents' coming to see their children as products of their will is outweighed by the fact that children could have increased well-being requires a variety of complex value judgments.

Even if scientists and engineers can appropriately provide relevant technical information about risks and benefits, they are not qualified to identify ethical and social values and to make judgments about how to best balance different values. They are unlikely to know enough about the public's values to be able to make risk decisions on their behalf; after all, the scientific and engineering community is scarcely representative of the general population. Moreover, evidence shows that social affiliations such as profession, gender, and political ideology influence what one determines to be a risk (Douglas and Wildavsky 1982). This explains, at least in part, why laypeople's and experts' views of risk are often different (Savadori et al. 2004). Laypeople tend to value both the content and the context of risk, whereas experts usually place greater emphasis on risk endpoints, such as human health hazards or toxicity levels, rather than the context in which risk might take place. Considerations about whether risks are imposed or voluntary, concerns about equitable distribution, questions about alternatives, and the thorny question of the trustworthiness of those in charge of imposing and managing risks are all relevant to risk determination and acceptance (Eiser, Miles, and Frewer 2002; Slovic 1998, 1999; Wynne 2001). Clearly, these are decisions that require public discussion and not just input from experts.

The problem is even more serious once it is recognized that values play a role not just in risk assessment but, as we have seen, in all aspects of technology development and application . Thus, if technologies embody specific values, either by design or via the norms necessary for their application, then democratic decisions about what such values should be are pertinent. If technologies mediate human actions, change the way we perceive and interact with reality, and shape, promote, and hinder particular moral values, then decisions about their development and implementation also call for democratic participation (Feenberg 2002; Sclove 1995; Shrader-Frechette 2007; Waelbers 2011).

Of course, practical issues about how to incorporate democratic processes into science and technology development and implementation are complex, and various proposals have been offered to ensure that democratic principles are not undermined in science and technology decision making. It is beyond the scope of this work to evaluate such proposals. My point here is to call attention to the fact that scientific and technological advances affect the kinds of societies we have and can develop and that these are questions that matter to everyone, not just to experts. A conception of science and technology as value-neutral illegitimately obfuscates the importance and legitimacy of citizens' participation in these vital issues.

Conclusion

Science and technology are not value-neutral activities. They embody particular values, shape and transform the world we live in, influence our practical options and our reasons for action, and affect what we take to be morally permissible or obligatory. If this is so, any evaluation of reprogenetic technologies that conceptualizes them as value-neutral or value-free is manifestly inadequate. Such a conceptualization certainly constitutes a mistaken description of these technologies and one that should be jettisoned. It also incorrectly limits the ethical evaluation of reprogenetics to an assessment of narrowly understood risks and potential benefits and therefore neglects other relevant normative concerns. It ignores so-called "soft impacts," such as the effects of reprogenetics on peoples' behavior, on the needs and expectations that people have of each other, or on moral values. It excludes any consideration about the values involved in the framing of our concerns, the meaning of our goals, the appropriateness of the means we adopt, and the relationship between means and ends. Equally problematic is the fact that a conception of science and technology as value-neutral renders democratic participation in scientific and technological policy making neither particularly useful nor pertinent.

But if proponents' assumption about the value-neutrality of science and technology is incorrect, then their analyses of the risks and benefits of using these technologies, even ones that find the benefits to outweigh the risks, fall short of providing a compelling ethical assessment of these techniques. They certainly fail to establish that we must pursue the development and implementation of reprogenetics. Moreover, ignoring the values that shape and are shaped by technological developments does not make those values disappear. What it does is conceal their presence and relevance, hindering critical scrutiny. Recognizing that science and technology in general, and reprogenetic technologies in particular, are not value-neutral allows us to unveil the values that influence and are influenced by reprogenetics and opens those values to critical examination.

References

Agar, Nicholas. 2005. *Liberal eugenics: in defence of human enhancement.* Malden, MA: Blackwell Publishing.

Anderson, Elizabeth. 2004. Uses of value judgments in science: a general argument, with lessons from a case study of feminist research on divorce. *Hypatia* 19 (1):1–24.

Asch, Adrienne. 1999. Prenatal diagnosis and selective abortion: a challenge to practice and policy. *American Journal of Public Health* 89 (11):1649–57.

———. 2003. Disability equality and prenatal testing: contradictory or compatible? *Florida State University Law Review* 30 (2):315–42.

Betz, Gregor. 2013. In defense of the value free ideal. *European Journal of the Philosophy of Science* 3 (2):207–20.

Bijker, Wiebe E., Thomas Parke Hughes, and T. J. Pinch. 1987. *The social construction of technological systems: new directions in the sociology and history of technology.* Cambridge, MA: MIT Press.

Birenbaum-Carmeli D. 2009. The politics of 'the natural family' in Israel: state policy and kinship ideologies. *Social Science & Medicine* 69: 1018–1024.

Borgmann, Albert. 1984. *Technology and the character of contemporary life: a philosophical inquiry.* Chicago: University of Chicago Press.

Bostrom, Nick. 2003. Human genetic enhancements: a transhumanist perspective. *Journal of Value Inquiry* 37 (4):493–506.

Brighouse, Harry, and Adam Swift. 2014. *Family values: the ethics of parent-child relationships.* Princeton, NJ: Princeton University Press.

Buchanan, Allen E. 2008. Enhancement and the ethics of development. *Kennedy Institute of Ethics Journal* 18 (1):1–34.

———. 2011. *Beyond humanity?: The ethics of biomedical enhancement.* Uehiro Series in Practical Ethics. New York: Oxford University Press.

Buchanan, Allen E., Dan W. Brock, Norman Daniels, and Daniel Wikler. 2000. *From chance to choice: genetics and justice.* New York: Cambridge University Press.

Bunge, Mario. 1966. Technology as applied science. *Technology and Culture* 7:329–47.

Callicott, J. B., L. B. Crowder, and K. Mumford. 1999. Current normative concepts in conservation. *Conservation Biology* 13 (1):22–35.

Chervenak, F. A., and L. B. McCullough. 1996. The fetus as a patient: an essential ethical concept for maternal-fetal medicine. *Journal of Maternal and Fetal Medicine* 5 (3):115–9.

Clarke, Adele. 2010. *Biomedicalization: technoscience, health, and illness in the U.S.* Durham, NC: Duke University Press.

Collins, Harry M. 1985. *Changing order: replication and induction in scientific practice.* Beverly Hills, CA: Sage Publications.

Conrad, Peter. 2007. *The medicalization of society: on the transformation of human conditions into treatable disorders.* Baltimore: Johns Hopkins University Press.

Crabb S, Augoustinos M. 2008. Genes and families in the media: implications of genetic discourse for constructions of the 'family'. *Health Sociology Review* 17: 303–312.

(CSDH) Commission on social determinants of health. 2008. *Closing the gap in a generation.* Geneva: World Health Organization & Commission on Social Determinants of Health.

Cuevas, Ana. 2005. The many faces of science and technology relationships. *Essays in Philosophy* 6 (1): Article 3.

Daniels, Norman. 2008. *Just health: meeting health needs fairly.* New York: Cambridge University Press.

Davis, Lennard J. 2013. *The disability studies reader.* 4th ed. New York: Routledge.

de Melo-Martin, Inmaculada. 2010. Defending human enhancement technologies: unveiling normativity. *Journal of Medical Ethics* 36 (8):483–7.

de Melo-Martin, Inmaculada, and Kristen Intemann. 2007. Can ethical reasoning contribute to better epidemiology?: a case study in research on racial health disparities. *European Journal of Epidemiology* 22 (4):215–21.

DeGrazia, David. 2012. *Creation ethics: reproduction, genetics, and quality of life.* New York: Oxford University Press.

Douglas, Heather. 2009. *Science, policy, and the value-free ideal.* Pittsburgh, PA: University of Pittsburgh Press.

Douglas, Mary, and Aaron B. Wildavsky. 1982. *Risk and culture: an essay on the selection of technical and environmental dangers.* Berkeley: University of California Press.

Duden, Barbara. 1993. *Disembodying women: perspectives on pregnancy and the unborn.* Cambridge, MA: Harvard University Press.

Dupré, John. 1993. *The disorder of things: metaphysical foundations of the disunity of science.* Cambridge, MA: Harvard University Press.

———. 2007. Fact and value. In *Value-free science?: ideals and illusions,* edited by H. Kincaid, J. Dupré, and A. Wylie. Oxford, UK: Oxford University Press.

Eiser, J. R., S. Miles, and L. J. Frewer. 2002. Trust, perceived risk, and attitudes toward food technologies. *Journal of Applied Social Psychology* 32 (11):2423–33.

Elliott, Kevin. 2009. The ethical significance of language in the environmental sciences: case studies from pollution research. *Ethics, Place, and Environment* 12 (2):157–73.

Fausto-Sterling, Anne. 1992. *Myths of gender: biological theories about women and men.* 2nd ed. New York: BasicBooks.

Feenberg, Andrew. 1999. *Questioning technology.* New York: Routledge.

———. 2002. *Transforming technology: a critical theory revisited.* New York: Oxford University Press.

Foucault, Michel. 2008. *The birth of biopolitics: lectures at the Collège de France, 1978–79.* New York: Palgrave Macmillan.

Froding, B., and M. Peterson. 2012. Why virtual friendship is no genuine friendship. *Ethics and Information Technology* 14 (3):201–7.

Green, Ronald Michael. 2007. *Babies by design: the ethics of genetic choice.* New Haven, CT: Yale University Press.

Haack, Susan. 1998. *Manifesto of a passionate moderate: unfashionable essays.* Chicago: University of Chicago Press.

Habermas, Jürgen. 1971. Technology and science as 'ideology.' In *Toward a rational society: student protest, science, and politics.* Boston: Beacon Press.

Haslanger Sally. 2009. Family, ancestry and self: what is the moral significance of biological ties? *Adoption & Culture* 2: 91–122.

Harding, Sandra G. 1998. *Is science multicultural?: postcolonialisms, feminisms, and epistemologies.* Race, Gender, and Science. Bloomington, IN: Indiana University Press.

Harris, John. 1998. Rights and reproductive choice. In *The Future of Human Reproduction*, edited by J. Harris and S. Holm. Oxford: Oxford University Press.

———. 2001. One principle and three fallacies of disability studies. *Journal of Medical Ethics* 27 (6):383–7.

———. 2005. Reproductive liberty, disease and disability. *Reproductive Biomedicine Online* 10 (suppl 1):13–6.

———. 2007. *Enhancing evolution: the ethical case for making better people.* Princeton, NJ: Princeton University Press.

———. 2015. Germline modification and the burden of human existence. *Cambridge Quarterly of Healthcare Ethics* 25 (1):6–18.

Herissone-Kelly, P. 2007a. Parental love and the ethics of sex selection. *Cambridge Quarterly of Healthcare Ethics* 16 (3):326–35.

———. 2007b. The "parental love" objection to nonmedical sex selection: deepening the argument. *Cambridge Quarterly of Healthcare Ethics* 16 (4):446–55.

Ihde, Don. 1990. *Technology and the lifeworld: from garden to earth.* Bloomington, IN: Indiana University Press.

———. 1993. *Postphenomenology.* Evanston, IL: Northwestern University Press.

Intemann, Kristen, and Inmaculada de Melo-Martin. 2010. Social values and scientific evidence: the case of the HPV vaccines. *Biology and Philosophy* 25 (2):203–13.

Irwin, Alan, and Brian Wynne. 1996. *Misunderstanding science?: the public reconstruction of science and technology.* New York: Cambridge University Press.

Jasanoff, Sheila. 1990. *The fifth branch: science advisers as policymakers.* Cambridge, MA: Harvard University Press.

———. 2004. *States of knowledge: the co-production of science and social order.* International Library of Sociology. London; New York: Routledge.

Jonas, Hans. 1984. *The imperative of responsibility: in search of an ethics for the technological age.* Chicago: University of Chicago Press.

Kass, Leon. 2002. *Life, liberty, and the defense of dignity: the challenge for bioethics.* 1st ed. San Francisco: Encounter Books.

Kitcher, Philip. 2001. *Science, truth, and democracy.* Oxford Studies in Philosophy of Science. New York: Oxford University Press.

Latour, Bruno. 1987. *Science in action: how to follow scientists and engineers through society.* Cambridge, MA: Harvard University Press.

———. 1993. *We have never been modern.* Cambridge, MA: Harvard University Press.

———. 1994. On technical mediation: philosophy, sociology, genealogy. *Common Knowledge* 3 (2):29–64.

———. 2005. *Reassembling the social: an introduction to actor-network-theory.* Clarendon Lectures in Management Studies. New York: Oxford University Press.

Lewontin, Richard C., Steven P. R. Rose, and Leon J. Kamin. 1984. *Not in our genes: biology, ideology, and human nature.* 1st ed. New York: Pantheon Books.

Lippman, A. 1992. Led (astray) by genetic maps: the cartography of the human genome and health care. *Social Science and Medicine* 35 (12):1469–76.

Lloyd, Elisabeth Anne. 2005. *The case of the female orgasm: bias in the science of evolution.* Cambridge, MA: Harvard University Press.

Longino, Helen E. 1990. *Science as social knowledge: values and objectivity in scientific inquiry.* Princeton, NJ: Princeton University Press.

———. 2002. *The fate of knowledge.* Princeton, NJ: Princeton University Press.

MacKenzie, Donald A., and Judy Wajcman. 1985. *The social shaping of technology: how the refrigerator got its hum.* Philadelphia: Open University Press.

Maienschein, J. 2002. Part II—what's in a name: embryos, clones, and stem cells. *American Journal of Bioethics* 2 (1):12–30.

Marmot, M., J. Allen, R. Bell, E. Bloomer, P. Goldblatt, and Consortium for the European review of social determinants of health and the health divide. 2012. WHO European review of social determinants of health and the health divide. Lancet 380 (9846):1011–29.

McDougall, R. 2005. Acting parentally: an argument against sex selection. *Journal of Medical Ethics* 31 (10):601–5.

Mitchell, Sandra. 2004. The prescribed and proscribed values in science policy. In *Science, Values and Objectivity*, edited by P. Machamer and G. Wolters. Pittsburgh, PA: University of Pittsburgh Press.

Nelkin, Dorothy, and M. Susan Lindee. 1995. *The DNA mystique: the gene as a cultural icon*. New York: Freeman.

Oyama, Susan. 1985. *The ontogeny of information: developmental systems and evolution*. New York: Cambridge University Press.

Parens, Erik. 2015. *Shaping our selves: on technology, flourishing, and a habit of thinking*. New York: Oxford University Press.

Parens, Erik, and Adrienne. Asch. 1999. The disability rights critique of prenatal genetic testing: reflections and recommendations. *Hastings Center Report* 29 (5).

Persson, I., and J. Savulescu. 2013. Getting moral enhancement right: the desirability of moral bioenhancement. *Bioethics* 27 (3):124–31.

Pitt, Joseph C. 2000. *Thinking about technology: foundations of the philosophy of technology*. New York: Seven Bridges Press.

Proctor, Robert, and Londa L. Schiebinger. 2008. *Agnotology: the making and unmaking of ignorance*. Stanford, CA: Stanford University Press.

Radder, Hans. 2009. Science, technology and the science-technology relationship. In *Philosophy of Technology and Engineering Sciences*, edited by A. Meijers. Amsterdam: North-Holland.

Rhodes, R. 1998. Genetic links, family ties, and social bonds: rights and responsibilities in the face of genetic knowledge. *Journal of Medical Philosophy* 23 (1):10–30.

Richardson, Sarah. 2012. Sexing the X: how the X became the 'female chromosome.' *Signs* 37 (4):909–33.

Robertson, John A. 1994. *Children of choice: freedom and the new reproductive technologies*. Princeton, NJ: Princeton University Press.

———. 2003. Procreative liberty in the era of genomics. *American Journal of Law and Medicine* 29 (4):439–87.

Roll-Hansen, Nils. 2005. *The Lysenko effect: the politics of science*. Amherst, N.Y.: Humanity Books.

Rose, Nikolas S. 2007. Politics of life itself: biomedicine, power, and subjectivity in the twenty-first century. Princeton, NJ: Princeton University Press.

Rothman, Barbara Katz. 1987. *The tentative pregnancy: prenatal diagnosis and the future of motherhood*. New York: Penguin Books.

Rudner, R. 1953. The scientist qua scientist makes value judgments. *Philosophy of Science* 20 (1):1–6.

Savadori, L., S. Savio, E. Nicotra, R. Rumiati, M. Finucane, and P. Slovic. 2004. Expert and public perception of risk from biotechnology. *Risk Analysis* 24 (5):1289–99.

Savulescu, Julian 1999. Sex selection: the case for. *Medical Journal of Australia* 171 (7):373–5.

———. 2001. Procreative beneficence: why we should select the best children. *Bioethics* 15 (5–6):413–26.

———. 2005. New breeds of humans: the moral obligation to enhance. *Reproductive Biomedicine Online* 10:36–9.

———. 2006. Justice, fairness, and enhancement. *Annals of the New York Academy of Sciences* 1093:321–38.

Savulescu, J., and E. Dahl. 2000. Sex selection and preimplantation diagnosis: a response to the Ethics Committee of the American Society of Reproductive Medicine. *Human Reproduction* 15 (9):1879–80.

Savulescu, J., and G. Kahane. 2009. The moral obligation to create children with the best chance of the best life. *Bioethics* 23 (5):274–90.

Savulescu, J., and I. Persson. 2012. Moral enhancement, freedom and the God machine. *Monist* 95 (3):399–421.

Savulescu, J., Jonathan Pugh, Thomas Douglas, and Christopher Gyngell. 2015. The moral imperative to continue gene editing research on human embryos. *Protein & Cell* 6 (7):476–9.

Sclove, Richard. 1995. *Democracy and technology*. The Conduct of Science Series. New York: Guilford Press.

Scully, Jackie Leach. 2008. *Disability bioethics: moral bodies, moral difference*. Feminist Constructions. Lanham, MD: Rowman & Littlefield.

Scully, Jackie Leach, T. Shakespeare, and S. Banks. 2006. Gift not commodity?: lay people deliberating social sex selection. *Sociology of Health and Illness* 28 (6):749–67.

Shrader-Frechette, Kristin. 1991. *Risk and rationality: philosophical foundations for populist reforms*. Berkeley: University of California Press.

———. 2007. *Taking action, saving lives: our duties to protect environmental and public health*. New York: Oxford University Press.

Silver, Lee M. 1997. *Remaking Eden: cloning and beyond in a brave new world.* 1st ed. New York: Avon Books.

Slovic, P. 1998. The risk game. *Reliability Engineering and System Safety* 59 (1):73–7.

———. 1999. Trust, emotion, sex, politics, and science: surveying the risk-assessment battlefield. [Reprinted from *Environment, Ethics, and Behavior*, edited by Bazerman, M. H., D. M. Messick, A. E. Tenbrunsel, and K. A. Wade-Benzoni. San Francisco: New Lexington, 1997:277–313.] *Risk Analysis* 19 (4):689–701.

Smith, K. R., S. Chan, and J. Harris. 2012. Human germline genetic modification: scientific and bioethical perspectives. *Archives of Medical Research* 43 (7):491–513.

Stangl, R. 2010. Selective terminations and respect for the disabled. *Journal of Medical Philosophy* 35 (1):32–45.

Swierstra, T., and K. Waelbers. 2012. Designing a good life: a matrix for the technological mediation of morality. *Science and Engineering Ethics* 18 (1):157–72.

Tabery, James. 2014. *Beyond versus: the struggle to understand the interaction of nature and nurture, life and mind.* Philosophical Issues in Biology and Psychology. Cambridge, MA: MIT Press.

Vallor, Shannon. 2012. Flourishing on Facebook: virtue friendship and new social media. *Ethics and Information Technology* 14 (3):185–199.

van de Poel, I. 2001. Investigating ethical issues in engineering design. *Science and Engineering Ethics* 7 (3):429–46.

Verbeek, Peter-Paul. 2005. *What things do: philosophical reflections on technology, agency, and design.* University Park, PA: Pennsylvania State University Press.

———. 2008. Obstetric ultrasound and the technological mediation of morality: a postphenomenological analysis. *Human Studies* 31 (1):11–26.

Waelbers, Katinka. 2011. *Doing good with technologies: taking responsibility for the social role of emerging technologies.* Philosophy of Engineering and Technology. New York: Springer.

Watson, Nick, Alan Roulstone, and Carol Thomas. 2012. *Routledge handbook of disability studies.* New York: Routledge.

Winner, Langdon. 1980. Do artifacts have politics? *Daedalus* 109 (1):121–36.

———. 1986. *The whale and the reactor: a search for limits in an age of high technology*. Chicago: University of Chicago Press.

Wynne, Brian. 2001. Creating public alienation: expert cultures of risk and ethics on GMOs. *Science and Culture (London)* 10 (4):445–81.

Zeiler K, Malmquist A. 2014. Lesbian shared biological motherhood: the ethics of IVF with reception of oocytes from partner. *Medicine Health Care and Philosophy* 17: 347–55.

Chapter 8

Enhancing the Assessment of Reprogenetic Technologies

The Case of Mitochondrial Replacement

Introduction

We saw in Chapter 2 that mitochondrial replacement techniques (MRTs), a new type of reproductive technology, aim to give women at risk of transmitting a mitochondrial disorder to their offspring the chance to have unaffected and genetically related children. Mitochondrial disorders can result from mutations in the mitochondrial DNA (mtDNA) or in the nuclear DNA (nDNA) and can affect people at different ages (Cree and Loi 2015; Lightowlers, Taylor, and Turnbull 2015; Wallace and Chalkia 2013). MRTs attempt to address disorders that result from mutated mtDNA. Pathology-causing mutations can be present in all of a person's mtDNA, or, more commonly, in a percentage of it. Evidence shows that the proportion of mutated mtDNA must exceed a critical threshold level before individuals are affected, with higher loads of mutated mtDNA usually correlating with more severe health problems. However, the percentage of mutant mtDNA varies significantly among individuals and even among organs and tissues within the same individual. This makes it difficult to predict whether a woman carrying mutated mtDNA will transmit a disease to her offspring as well as the severity of the disease if it is transmitted. Sometimes, asymptomatic women with low levels of mutated mtDNA have children with high levels of mutated mtDNA who are affected by mitochondrial disorders. And it is possible for a phenotypically healthy mother harboring 50% of mutated mtDNA to produce both healthy and severely affected children (Burgstaller, Johnston, and Poulton 2015).

MRTs are qualitatively different from other existent reprogenetic technologies for two reasons. First, because mitochondria have their own genome, embryos created through these technologies contain three different sources of DNA: the usual nDNA from both prospective parents and the mtDNA from the woman who provides the eggs with unaffected mitochondria (Amato et al. 2014). Second, because mtDNA is maternally inherited, males created through these technologies will inherit the three sources of DNA but will not pass mtDNA on to their offspring, whereas females will transmit mtDNA mutations to subsequent generations. MRTs thus involve germline modifications. In October of 2015, the United Kingdom approved the use of these new techniques and thus became the first country to explicitly legalize germline modifications (HFE 2015). However, regulations still need to be developed to evaluate applications from physicians who want to use MRTs in the clinic (HFEA 2015).

As usual, proponents of reprogenetic technologies have been quick both to dismiss criticisms and to embrace these techniques enthusiastically. In Harris' words:

> There is a large degree of desperation and not a little callousness in the objections that have been made so far to mitochondrial donation. This procedure—which will pave the way to helping some 2,500 women in the U.K. have children related to them and avoid some terrible diseases—is,

I believe, to be unreservedly welcomed. Unfortunately, some people seem to object regardless of the evidence and are willing to defend absurdly high standards of safety, standards that are not met by normal sexual reproduction, let alone by ARTs [assisted reproductive technologies] (Harris 2015b, 5).

For reprogenetics proponents, MRTs serve an important need, have been shown to be safe enough, and, at least in countries like the United Kingdom with a sophisticated regulatory system for reprogenetics, present no other problems that would call for prohibition or a moratorium at this time. Nonetheless, and as has been the case with other reprogenetic technologies, the ethical assessments of MRTs by proponents of reprogenetics leave much to be desired. They focus on a narrow set of concerns, inappropriately neglect the uncertainties surrounding these technologies, and ignore important normative considerations. This chapter presents a feminist analysis of MRTs, one that takes into account the social context in which they will be implemented, attends to more than simply risks and benefits narrowly understood, and addresses the value-laden nature of these technologies. As we will see, an evaluation that conceptualizes MRTs as more than mere value-neutral tools calls into question the moral permissibility of these technologies.

Reprogenetics Proponents' Assessments of Mitochondrial Replacement Techniques

Characteristically, reprogenetics advocates' evaluations of MRTs focus on risks and possible benefits narrowly understood. They appropriately call attention to the potential benefits of these technologies. Although the burden of mitochondrial disorders is difficult to calculate because of the marked variation in their clinical features, these disorders can cause significant suffering and premature death (Lightowlers, Taylor, and Turnbull 2015). Therapy for mitochondrial diseases is inadequate and mostly palliative. Their prevalence is also difficult to establish because of clinical and genetic heterogeneity. In a recent study, however, researchers calculated that the average number of births per year among women at risk of transmitting serious mtDNA disease is 152 in the United Kingdom and 778 in the United States (Gorman et al. 2015).

Of course, potential benefits need to be balanced against safety considerations. For proponents, these safety considerations have been appropriately addressed. Indeed, Harris (2015b, 5) agrees that, as far as safety is concerned, these technologies are now good to go. He believes that, given the balance of risks and benefits, MRTs are safe enough for use in human beings. What other risks do proponents entertain? Harris considers concerns that children born through MRTs might suffer psychologically because they would have "three genetic parents." To him, such fears seem overblown for several reasons. First, he considers the "three genetic parents" label to be completely inappropriate because he takes the contribution of the mtDNA to be minute and not affecting "any of the traits that confer the usual family resemblances and distinctive personal features in which both parents and children are interested" (Harris 2015b, 6). Second, he dismisses this concern because he judges, I think correctly, that a genetic contribution is neither necessary nor sufficient for parenthood. Although it might be the case that a child could be confused if told she has three parents, Harris believes that the child is likely to be happier than she would have been given the alternative: to suffer from a mitochondrial disease. Indeed, for Harris, if someone "were condemned unnecessarily to a life of pain and illness, [that person] would really have something to complain of, and indeed somebody to blame. And among those somebodies to blame would be anyone who opposes the introduction of this new technology" (Harris 2015b, 7).

Harris also contemplates, and discards, another risk presented by critics of MRTs. Some argue that individuals have a right to know their genetic origins and, consequently, that individuals created through MRTs have a right to know the identity of the woman who provided the mitochondria. For Harris (2015b, 7), however, the phenomenon of non-paternity makes this alleged right to know "dangerous nonsense," and he maintains that nothing good can come of recognizing a right to know or a duty to disclose genetic origins.

Finally, Harris (2015b) addresses objections to MRTs that result from the fact that children and future generations cannot consent to these interventions. He, of course, acknowledges that given the fact that these individuals do not yet exist, they simply cannot provide consent. But he believes this to be ethically unproblematic. After all, prospective parents and actual parents make decisions on behalf of their unborn and born children routinely without asking for their consent, and presumably we consider these practices to be ethically appropriate. He also believes that, in any case, were the children and future generations resulting from MRTs to be asked to consent, they would be happy to do so given the benefits to their health that these technologies presumably entail.

According to this (not particularly persuasive) assessment of the risks and benefits of MRTs, there are no reasons to stall their use in human beings. Indeed, as the quote at the beginning shows, Harris (2015b) actually considers that MRTs should be unreservedly welcomed. In what follows, however, I offer what I take to be a more ethically robust evaluation of these techniques. I begin by assessing existent evidence regarding the potential benefits and safety of MRTs. I then discuss other relevant normative considerations that proponents of reprogenetics ignore. I do not claim this to be an exhaustive assessment of MRTs; many other factors might be of relevance in determining the moral permissibility of these technologies. Arguably, however, the factors I discuss here are essential to an appropriate evaluation of MRTs and therefore should not be excluded.

On Risks and Benefits

As I showed in Chapter 7, proponents' assessments of risks and potential benefits, even when correctly done, fail to establish the ethical appropriateness of developing and implementing particular technological innovations because they leave out other pertinent considerations. Nonetheless, and again not unlike their evaluations of other reprogenetic technologies, even the narrow risk-benefit analysis they provide is problematic.

Let us begin by considering the potential benefits of MRTs. Two things seem relevant in this respect. One is the number of people who will be helped by these technologies. As indicated earlier, about 150 women in the United Kingdom and almost 800 in the United States could benefit yearly from MRTs. Although the ability to reduce the burden of mitochondrial disorders is, of course, an important benefit, these numbers are relatively small. Although this alone is insufficient reason not to develop and implement these technologies, it is certainly something to take into account. In any case, the number of beneficiaries is likely to be smaller than estimated. This is so because many of these women might not want to undergo the risks involved in in vitro fertilization (IVF) and might also be unwilling to expose their future children to unknown risks. Because of the expenses involved, the risks, and the fact that the effects of mitochondrial diseases are quite variable, others might consider alternatives to these technologies. For instance, they might decide to have children without assistance. In fact, some might be reluctant to become pregnant at all, given that women suffering from at least some mitochondrial diseases might be at higher risk of complications during pregnancy and labor (Say et al. 2011).

One could argue that I have minimized the potential benefits that MRTs can produce. After all, although these technologies are being developed to help women with some types of mitochondrial diseases, other women could also benefit from their use. For instance, some evidence suggests that declining oocyte quality, rather than simply reduced ovarian reserve, is an important factor in age-related infertility (Tatone 2008). According to this evidence, although such decline might result from a variety of factors, cytoplasmic deficiencies are related to problems in chromosome segregation and may affect embryonic development before implantation (Tatone 2008). Similarly, some contend that increased mtDNA mutations resulting from age and other types of mitochondrial dysfunction may be involved in age-related infertility (Bentov and Casper 2013). MRTs might theoretically solve these problems by permitting use of the cytoplasmic content of eggs from younger women. MRTs have thus been proposed as a way to alleviate age-related infertility while allowing women to have genetically related offspring (Wolf, Mitalipov, and Mitalipov 2015). Given cultural and social changes that contribute to more and more women having children at a later age, and assuming that MRTs are an effective solution to age-related infertility, the number who could use these technologies might be significantly greater than the number of women suffering from some mitochondrial diseases.

This seems correct, and if the history of reproductive and reprogenetic technologies is any indication, and again assuming that MRTs could solve age-related infertility, the use of these techniques will likely be expanded to such cases. As we saw in Chapter 2, IVF was initially introduced to help women with blocked fallopian tubes, but the indications for its use expanded rapidly (Zhao et al. 2011). Similarly, although intracytoplasmic sperm injection (ICSI) was pioneered as a way to address severe male factor infertility, it accounts today for 70% to 80% of all IVF cycles performed (Rubino et al. 2016). Oocyte cryopreservation, advanced originally as an option for women who were undergoing cancer treatment, is today advertised to young women who want to preserve the option of having genetically related children at a later date (Cil and Seli 2013).

Although the fact that more women could use MRTs might be thought of as an added benefit, it is not clear that it should be so deemed. In fact, good reasons can be provided that render this very likely possibility a risk rather than a benefit. Reprogenetic technologies have become routine medical practice in spite of the absence of evidence on long-term safety outcomes (Braude and Khalaf 2013; Dondorp and de Wert 2011; Evers 2013). More women using MRTs simply means more women undergoing unknown risks to themselves and their offspring as well as unknown effects on future generations. Furthermore, infertility related to trying to have children at a later age is not a medical problem but a social one. If medical technologies, with the agreement of the medical profession, are going to be used to address these social problems, the social consequences of such use should also be considered. After all, presenting age-related infertility as a free choice that women make is misleading. Such choice is the result of social and institutional practices that make it difficult for women who want to work or pursue an education to do so and have children at a younger age. Rather than enhance women's choices in a meaningful way, the use of MRTs to solve age-related infertility simply normalizes the social injustices that force many women to choose between a career and raising children.

A second important consideration when evaluating the potential benefits of MRTs is whether their use will in fact prevent transmission of mitochondrial disorders in human beings. At this point, the answer is unknown, given that the techniques have not been used to create children.[1] It is true that the laboratory evidence is promising, with minimal amounts of mtDNA carryover (Amato et al. 2014). However, both spindle transfer and pronuclear transfer are associated with some degree of mtDNA carryover, and thus with possible transmission of mutated mtDNA to the embryo. Evidence suggests that the amount of mutant mtDNA transferred is insufficient to cause disease in the resulting child (Smeets et al. 2015). Nevertheless, the fact that some mutated mtDNA can be transferred is relevant for the success of MRTs. Evidence from animal studies suggests that preferential replication of mutant mtDNA could exist (Burgstaller, Johnston, and Poulton 2015). If mutant mtDNA proliferates over healthy mtDNA, it will be amplified during development and during the lifetime of the offspring. If so, this phenomenon would limit the effectiveness of MRTs. Some evidence with animals shows that haplotype matching of the donor and the recipient might ameliorate some of these concerns (Burgstaller, Johnston, and Poulton 2015), but it is not known whether this would be the case also in humans.

What about safety concerns related to MRTs? MRTs require the use of IVF, so the risks associated with that technique will

---

1. A technique called cytoplasmic or ooplasmic transfer was briefly used in some clinics during the late 1990s and until 2001. In 2001, the US Food and Drug Administration (FDA) concerned about safety, intervened, requiring fertility clinics to submit requests for approval before any other patient could be treated. No request was submitted. Some estimate that about 30 children have been born worldwide through this procedure (Barritt et al. 2001). Cytoplasmic transfer, however, is different from mitochondrial transfer. Cytoplasmic transfer, consists in transferring the partical cytoplasm content of a healthy donor egg into the oocyte of an infertile woman. A child resulting from this technique will inherit all of the mother's mtDNA and some of the donor's mtDNA. As we have seen, in mitochondrial transfer the goal is to eliminate all of the mtDNA from the prospective mother's egg and create embryos that contain primarily mtDNA from the healthy donor egg.

also be present for women who undergo MRTs. Also present are the risks to women providing the eggs necessary for MRTs. In fact, more women will be put at risk when using these technologies. In studies evaluating the feasibility of spindle transfer, for instance, more than half of the reconstructed eggs that were fertilized showed abnormal development (Tachibana et al. 2013). It is conceivable that MRTs could also affect implantation rates, which would ultimately require even more women to undergo the risks associated with egg procurement.

Qualitative differences between MRTs and currently used reprogenetic technologies make comparisons of safety profiles inadequate when assessing risks. Other reprogenetic technologies used today do not involve the introduction of a third-party source of DNA, and they do not produce alterations that are transmissible to future generations. This does not mean that any technology that creates germline modifications should, simply by virtue of that fact, be prohibited. It does mean, however, that the uncertainties involved in this type of research are significant and that those affected by such uncertainties include not only the individuals created by the manipulated embryos but also future generations. Surely these are important areas of concern.

Of note also is the fact that clinical use of reprogenetic technologies before careful evaluation of their safety is not at all uncommon. As indicated earlier, reproductive technologies in general have routinely been brought to clinical practice without preclinical studies or clinical trials (Braude and Khalaf 2013; Dondorp and de Wert 2011; Evers 2013). It is true that other medical interventions (e.g., some surgeries) have also been introduced in the clinic without rigorous preclinical and clinical safety studies. However, often those interventions have involved life-threatening conditions for which other options are not available or are inadequate.[2] Reprogenetic technologies are not life-saving techniques. Granted, MRTs have received more scientific scrutiny than other reproductive and reprogenetic technologies, but given the inadequate long-term safety testing of many of these technologies, we should be wary of using other reprogenetic technologies as the standard of safety. Moreover, as I have indicated, MRTs are significantly different from currently employed reprogenetic technologies, making the use of such a standard even less appropriate.

Importantly, life-saving biomedical interventions characteristically follow strict preclinical and clinical study requirements before they become clinical practice. Whether or not these strict requirements should also be the standard for reprogenetic interventions, it seems clear that introducing MRTs in the clinic based only on the existent evidence, as the United Kingdom might be doing soon enough, calls for justification. Surely, no matter how much support these technologies draw from women and families affected by mitochondrial disorders, it cannot be any stronger than the support that potentially life-saving interventions attract from people affected by life-threatening diseases.

MRTs have been used in mice (Wang et al. 2014) and in monkeys (Tachibana et al. 2009), and although offspring have not until now shown obvious health problems, inferences from animal models to human beings should be made with caution. There is significant evidence that clearly encouraging results encountered in studies with animal models often fail to translate into efficacy in clinical studies (Begley and Ellis 2012; Hackam and Redelmeier 2006; Perel et al. 2007). Although the biology of

---

2. Of course, insofar as the medical procedures in question are elective, their introduction in the clinic without appropriate evidence also constitutes a problem. It hardly needs to be argued that the fact that some problematic practices already exist is not a good reason to add more of them.

human beings shares many commonalities with that of rodents and nonhuman primates, inferences from animal models to human beings are fraught with difficulties. In fact, the results of maternal spindle transfer in monkeys were not predictive of the results with human eggs (Tachibana et al. 2013; Tachibana, et al. 2009). In monkeys, reconstructed embryos resulted in blastocyst development and quality comparable to those of controls, and this was true also for the derivation of embryonic stem cell lines. However, although reconstructed human eggs showed similar fertilization rates as controls, more than half of the fertilized eggs had abnormal fertilization. Furthermore, there were differences between treatment and control groups in the isolation rate of embryonic stem cells (Morrow et al. 2015). Of course, the fact that results from animal studies are not always good predictors of human outcomes does not mean that animal studies are useless, but care should be taken not to draw overly confident conclusions from such studies in regard to human beings, particularly when the inferences result from a limited number of animal models.

Long-term safety studies of MRTs have not been conducted in animals, and questions about various safety considerations remain. For instance, knowledge about the consequences of epigenetic effects resulting from the multiple embryo manipulations that take place with reprogenetic technologies is still poor (Calle et al. 2012; Kohda 2013). Significant uncertainties also exist regarding the impact of the interactions among different DNA sources. Some have signaled that interactions between different mtDNAs—the one coming from the healthy mitochondria and the one that may be carried over from the prospective mother's egg—might have negative effects on the offspring (Sharpley et al. 2012). Whether or not the low levels of carryover resulting from MRTs will be sufficient to eliminate these problems is unknown.

Some contend that extensive evidence exists that the interactions between mtDNA and nDNA are important in determining health outcomes, both in humans and in other species (Morrow et al. 2015). They have cautioned that the mismatch between nDNA and donor mtDNA might produce unintended and unanticipated effects due to the co-evolution of nuclear and mitochondrial genomes (Dobler et al. 2014; Dunham-Snary and Ballinger 2015; Morrow et al. 2015). Because of the critical importance of energy conversion, for which mitochondrial function is vital, natural selection is likely to have exerted significant evolutionary pressure on genomic combinations of mtDNA with nDNA. The mismatch between them resulting from MRTs might affect the phenotypic expression of various traits that are fundamental to the life history of individuals and species, such as reproductive success, aging, and metabolic functioning. Given that MRTs affect not only the children born through these technologies but also future generations, concerns about evolutionary effects are of particular significance. Researchers have also called attention to the fact that studies done to evaluate the feasibility of MRTs were not designed to test for incompatibilities between nuclear and mitochondrial genomes and therefore cannot be used to predict the population-wide likelihood of incompatibilities after the use of MRTs (Morrow et al. 2015).

Of course, all new biomedical interventions involve some degree of uncertainty about short-term and especially long-term impacts. But that does not seem to be a good reason to fail to reduce such uncertainties if possible. In spite of the contention by proponents of reprogenetics that uncertainties are present in other biomedical interventions (Harris 2015b), this is clearly not a good reason to overconfidently declare that the risks and uncertainties of MRTs should not worry us excessively. Furthermore, considerations about the existence of uncertainties, both known and unknown, are important not just because they mean that we lack knowledge relevant to the women who will be using MRTs, the children who will be born through their use, and future generations. The presence of uncertainties is also important for other reasons that have ethical import (Jonas 1984; Wynne 2001). As I discussed in Chapter 7, the degree of uncertainty that one is open to tolerate involves complex normative judgments that include a variety of factors such as the potential benefits achieved, trust in the scientific community and in the institutions that are in charge of managing risks and uncertainties, and the existence of alternatives to realize similar legitimate ends. It is ethically problematic to systematically evade discussions about the possibility that even the best scientific data and the best assessments may be limited. In the case of MRTs, such data are at best scarce, and at worst, nonexistent. If considerations about known and unknown uncertainties are dismissed and excluded from debate, it is unlikely that institutional regulations and safety mechanisms will be put into practice to appropriately deal with unknown consequences. Furthermore, if uncertainties are neglected, necessary research to reduce them is unlikely to be conducted. When these concerns are taken into account, and recognizing that all interventions require judgments about whether they are "safe enough" rather than about whether they are completely safe, it is at least not obvious that current evidence should lead us to assert that MRTs are safe enough, as proponents of reprogenetics insist (Harris 2015a, 2015b).

One might object that judgments about whether these technologies are indeed safe enough should be left to those concerned. As Harris (2015b) reminds us, "sometimes this decision must be left to those who wish to use the procedure and on whom the risk falls." Although allowing people who will run the risks to determine what is safe enough for them is often an appropriate strategy, there are a variety of problems with it in this case. First, clearly we do not proceed in such a manner when conducting biomedical research in human beings. Regulations for the protection of human subjects simply prevent individuals who might well wish to run the risks resulting from research participation to determine whether certain interventions are safe enough for them. That is the task of review committees, which in fact exist to assess whether research interventions are actually "safe enough" to be used in humans. And this is the case even with potentially life-saving medical procedures. Of course, once the interventions in question have been declared "safe enough" by others, and usually after a rigorous preclinical research process, those on whom the risks will fall are free to decide whether they find those risks, on balance, acceptable. But determinations about whether the interventions are safe enough for them to accept those risks are left to others, appropriately so for a variety of reasons (Bender, Flicker, and Rhodes 2007; Leonard 2009).

Second, even if one were to agree that only those who run the risks should be determining what constitutes "safe enough," more is needed to determine the relevant "who." If the only risks that are of concern are health hazards, then MRT risks fall on several parties: the women who will be using these procedures; the women who will provide the eggs necessary for both research and clinical use of these new technologies; the offspring whose health might be affected by the embryo manipulations; and future generations of individuals who might also be negatively affected by the behavior of mtDNA. Certainly, neither the offspring nor future generations can provide consent, and although this might ultimately fail as an objection to the use of these technologies, it is important to point out that "those on whom the risks fall" and those "who wish to use the procedures" are not one and the same.

Third, even if we restrict our concerns to those who can in fact consent, it is not clear that the consent that could be given would be a valid one. After all, the issue at stake is whether there is enough appropriate information about risks to women undergoing the procedures and to their offspring and whether the uncertainties, both known and unknown, are such that they challenge the possibility of an autonomous authorization. Even if clinicians providing MRT services are conscientious individuals offering all existing information to their patients, the problem still remains that the data are, at least at this point, inadequate. Let us not forget that these will be first-in-human experiments and that the preclinical evidence involves a very limited number of animal models as well as limited follow-up time. Moreover, given the publicity these technologies have received, their presentation as a "miracle cure" for at least some types of mitochondrial disorders, and the usual underplay of both known and unknown uncertainties in these discussions, it is not unreasonable to at least call attention to the difficulties of providing a truly informed consent under these circumstances. Some evidence suggests that women who use reprogenetic technologies lack adequate information to make informed decisions, adding to these concerns (Stewart et al. 2001). This does not mean that it is impossible to give an informed consent under conditions of uncertainty. Conceivably, appropriate information could be provided to people concerning the degree of ignorance, what information is lacking, the importance of the information that is missing, and the many unknown unknowns—which in the case of MRTs are many indeed. However, because these technologies are simply presented as not unsafe, and given the usual disregard of long-term risks and uncertainties in the field of reproductive technologies and reprogenetics, it is not clear that the consent of women undergoing these procedures should be seen as beyond dispute. Importantly, this is not a claim about women's ability to make autonomous decisions. It is a claim about the conditions necessary for someone to be able to make such decisions.

Directing concerns about the safety of MRTs to the consent of women using these procedures simply distracts from the inadequacy of such conditions.

Likewise, although more is known about risks to the women providing the eggs that will be needed for MRTs, we saw in Chapter 6 that there is a significant lack of data about long-term risks to their health. Here again, evidence suggests that current practices, both in countries with strict regulations and in those where such regulations are lenient, present challenges to women's ability to give a truly informed consent when providing their eggs (Keehn et al. 2015; Uroz and Guerra 2009). That MRTs might call for a considerable number of egg donors because of their inefficiency in producing viable embryos (Tachibana et al. 2013) is all the more concerning.

Fourth, technological interventions usually affect individuals other than those using the technologies in question and who also have the ability to consent. It is true that those impacts might well not be health related. But it is simply incorrect to assume that health effects are the only relevant considerations when assessing reprogenetic technologies. If MRTs have other impacts (and, as shown later, they surely do) that go beyond the health consequences to those using them—such as effects on values that we might want to preserve or jettison, on women's status, or on research funding—then it is unclear why the decisions about whether the technologies in question are safe enough should be left only to those who will use them.

It seems, therefore, that to claim at this point that MRTs are "safe enough" to be used in human beings is an overstatement. This is the case because one is defending not "absurdly high standards of safety" (Harris 2015b, 5) but the kinds of standards that we defend for most other biomedical interventions, even those that are directed to life-threatening conditions. Clearly, if saving someone's life is not sufficient to lower standards of evidence and safety, compelling reasons should be given for why we should lower them when no life is at stake.

Broadening Risk Assessment Considerations

Although concerns about safety call into question the moral appropriateness of using these technologies in human beings at this point, I have argued in prior chapters that safety issues are not the only relevant factors when assessing new technological innovations. Here, I tackle some of the other normative considerations that are pertinent to the ethical evaluation of MRTs. Attention to them also disputes conclusions that MRTs are morally permissible.

Assessing the Ends of Mitochondrial Replacement Techniques

In Chapter 7, I argued that considerations about the ends that new technologies aim to achieve, what the value of such ends might be, and whether the innovations in question constitute appropriate means to realizing desired ends are essential to any ethical evaluation of new technological innovations. How do MRTs fare in regard to these issues?

What is the goal that MRTs aim to attain? These technologies are not uncommonly presented as a way to reduce the burdens of mitochondrial diseases. As mentioned earlier, these disorders can cause significant pain and suffering, so few would deny that this is a worthy goal. Nonetheless, this characterization is only partially correct. In fact, insofar as this is the goal of MRTs, they are not a particularly effective means to achieve such an aim. Assuming that MRTs will actually be effective in limiting the transmission of mitochondrial diseases, their contribution to reducing the burdens of these disorders does not result from their ability to alleviate the suffering of any existing affected individual. That is, MRTs are not a treatment. What they might be able to do is reduce or eliminate the possibility that some individuals will be born with these disorders. This, of course, can still be a very good thing, a goal that many would find valuable. However, if other means currently exist that are less risky, less costly, and afford additional benefits, arguably such means should be given priority. And it turns out that such alternatives actually do exist.

First, and most obviously, prospective parents can adopt a child.[3] Millions of children who need good homes exist in the world. Adoption would not only help women with mitochondrial disorders become mothers without risking transmission of such disorders, but would also have the benefit of placing children in environments more conducive to their flourishing. Although it is true that adoption can be expensive and time-consuming, these costs are unlikely to fare poorly when contrasted with those of undergoing MRTs. These technologies, which involve the use of IVF, are not cheap. IVF itself is relatively inefficient, and the process of obtaining embryos with MRTs might make the pregnancy rates for these techniques—at least initially—lower than usual for IVF outcomes. I will say more about this alternative later. For now, it is sufficient to note that a safe, highly beneficial alternative exists for women with mitochondrial disorders who want to become mothers and avoid the transmission of these disorders.

Second, these women can use eggs from other, unaffected women. This alternative has the advantage over adoption of allowing women to experience pregnancy, although it requires putting those women who provide the eggs at risk with no direct

---

3. I am not suggesting that adoption is an easy process. This concern is discussed further in a later section.

benefit to themselves. Granted, the availability of eggs is limited, but this problem affects not only the alternative I am proposing but also MRTs themselves. Indeed, it constitutes a more serious problem for MRTs because the manipulations required to obtain unaffected embryos appear to affect the viability of the resulting embryos. As I indicated earlier, in experiments to demonstrate the feasibility of MRTs, more than half of the viable eggs used for spindle transfer showed abnormal fertilization (Tachibana, et al. 2013). For this reason, MRTs will require many more eggs and thus put many more women at risk to obtain the same number of viable embryos as egg donation procedures now produce. If MRTs turn out to affect implantation rates, even more eggs will be needed.

Moreover, if reduction of the burdens of mitochondrial disorders were indeed the goal, basic and clinical studies of the causes of these diseases, as well as other preventive and treatment strategies, would in all likelihood be more effective than research on MRTs. After all, even if all the women who could be eligible to use them did so—a big "if" indeed—these technologies would have a relatively limited application. On the other hand, research on the mitochondrial disorders themselves and on more effective treatments for them would be of use to all of those suffering from these diseases. Let us not forget that funding for any scientific and technological program has opportunity costs, and that decisions about resource distribution should take into account how to obtain the best results in the most efficient ways. By this account, MRTs are unlikely to be the wisest of choices.

So, insofar as MRTs are means to achieving what many would consider a legitimate and very worthy goal (i.e., reducing the burdens of mitochondrial diseases), they are not particularly good means of realizing such an end, and more effective means already exist. The goal for which MRTs are a more appropriate means is more precisely characterized as that of allowing women who are at risk of transmitting mitochondrial disorders to have unaffected and *genetically related* offspring. Understood in this way, neither adoption nor the use of donated eggs constitutes an appropriate alternative because neither of them preserves a genetic connection between the prospective mother and the offspring.

Still, women at risk of passing on mitochondrial diseases who wish to have unaffected, genetically related offspring do have other existent alternatives. For instance, they can use preimplantation genetic diagnosis (PGD) to select the embryos that have a below-the-threshold level of mutated mtDNA (Smeets et al. 2015). Indeed, PGD has been successfully used for individuals with some mtDNA mutations (Sallevelt et al. 2013). It is true that this method, even if effective in some instances, would be of no help in cases in which the level of mutated mtDNA is very high. Such cases, however, appear to be relatively uncommon (Smeets et al. 2015).

More importantly, although the ability to have genetically related offspring is highly valued by many people, it is implausible to argue that satisfying such desire should constitute a scientific priority given the many pressing needs that exist. Although strong and persuasive arguments can be given for the goods of parenting (Brighouse and Swift 2014), few would argue that a genetic connection is a necessary condition for those goods. Were we living in a world of unlimited resources, it would make sense to attend not only to people's needs but to their legitimate desires. But I hardly need to point out that we do not live in such a world.

Furthermore, if the ability of women to have healthy and genetically related children is indeed the goal, then safe and often cheap alternatives already exist that can help accomplish this goal much more efficiently than MRTs can. For instance, a recent evaluation of the Millennium Development Goals for maternal and child health reported that 17,000 children die every day from preventable causes, and millions of women die or suffer from acute or chronic illnesses related to childbirth (Requejo and Bhutta 2015). The report also indicated that effective preventive and treatment interventions exist for reproductive, maternal, newborn, and child care. And although most cases of maternal and child mortality and morbidity occur in developing nations, the problem also exists in industrialized countries. In particular, both the United Kingdom, where MRTs have been legalized, and the United States, where such legalization is under consideration, have some of the worst child mortality rates among Western industrialized nations (Taylor et al. 2015). Investment in basic and applied research on pregnancy and infancy would thus go significantly further than investment in the development of MRTs to achieve the goal of permitting women to have healthy and genetically related offspring. In the United Kingdom, for instance, evidence indicates that less than 5% of total research funding from public and charitable sources is directed toward child health (Taylor et al. 2015). Spending commensurate with the burdens of maternal and child morbidity and mortality could allow many more women to enjoy the benefits of having healthier and genetically related offspring. Needless to say, such investments would have additional benefits that are lacking in the case of MRTs. After all, funding for these alternatives is likely to benefit members of the population who are already marginalized, and thus their effects on the well-being of those individuals and of society as a whole is bound to be much more significant. We would do well to remember that scientific and technological benefits should accrue to all members of the public. Science and technology are, not incidentally, public goods.

Insofar as MRTs are proposed also as a solution to age-related infertility, similar considerations apply. Women in this situation have other options to become mothers, and thus the precise goal of MRTs is simply to allow women to have genetically related off-spring. That women today tend to have children at a later point in their lives is the result of particular social and institutional practices that make it challenging for women to both pursue successful careers and have children at a younger age. The introduction of MRTs does nothing to solve these real obstacles and at the same time normalizes problematic social practices.

Of course, reprogenetics proponents might be sympathetic to these concerns. They might nonetheless argue that insofar as the use of these technologies is funded by patients, claims about the opportunity costs for other potential research projects and treatments are of little interest. But this seems incorrect. Even in the United States, where access to reprogenetic technologies is mostly based on people's ability to pay, some insurance companies cover some of these procedures. In countries with national care systems, such as the United Kingdom, access to these technologies is covered for at least some individuals. Furthermore, research to develop MRTs may receive public funds that will then not be available for other projects. Excluding the very unlikely scenario in which such funding is called into being only by the possibility of its being used for MRTs, and even if the funding for these technologies were completely private, opportunity costs still exist because again such funding will not be available for other research programs.

In any case, claims that opportunity cost considerations are of little relevance when MRTs are mostly funded by patients also ignores the fact that the direction of research can be affected in ways that ultimately result in opportunity costs. For instance, even if only private resources were used to develop and implement MRTs, focus on this type of research might lead scientists away from other, more effective alternatives. Furthermore, training of researchers involves the use of public resources, so their subsequent use purely for privately funded research can still be seen as involving the diversion of public funds. Finally, the use of MRTs, even if paid for completely out of pocket, can still have effects on public funds in various ways. Ensuring follow-up of children born through MRTs to assess their health and well-being will surely fall on government agencies. Excess costs to health care systems could also result from the increased use of services by women who use MRTs and their children. In summary, even in the unlikely scenario in which no public funding is used for the development or use of MRTs, opportunity costs would still be created.

Proponents of MRTs might also object that the more effective alternatives that I have proposed require challenging and perhaps unattainable institutional changes. They could argue that allocating funds for preventive measures is less appealing than doing so for MRTs because the latter fulfills the needs (or strong desires) of identifiable people, whereas the former helps people who are unidentified others. Similarly, proponents might counter that global economic pressures make it difficult to provide the necessary means to care for the health of the millions of mothers and children who could benefit and that my proposals for improving the health and well-being of mothers and their genetically related offspring might require an extensive period of time before results are obtained. Likewise, institutional changes to practices that make it difficult for women to have careers and children at a younger age would likely be difficult to accomplish.

There are several problems with these responses, however. First, even when the objection calls appropriate attention to the difficulties of social and institutional changes, this should hardly lead anyone to conclude, as Harris (2015b) does, that MRTs ought to be unreservedly welcomed. On the contrary, insofar as these statements are correct, dispirited resignation would be a more appropriate attitude. After all, it is clear that better means exist to achieve the ends that these new reprogenetic technologies presumably set out to achieve. That the development of these technologies nevertheless appears inevitable (Baylis 2013) and that other, more effective means will fail to be implemented does not seem to be a reason for rejoicing.

Second, the unreserved embrace of these technologies is unlikely to contribute to changing the status quo. Thus, evaluations of new reprogenetic technologies that simply assume that other, better alternatives are impracticable become a self-fulling prophecy, sanctioning current conditions without any objections. In fact, if half of the ink that proponents have spilled rejecting arguments against reprogenetic technologies had been directed to calling attention to the mismatch between goals and the means to achieve them, perhaps alternative and more effective means would not appear so difficult and unattainable. At the very least, it would be clear that rejecting the development and implementation of MRTs is the result not of obscure arguments about the value of the unmanipulated human genome, fears about the implications of three-parent children, or concerns about the alleged right to know one's genetic origins but of the desire to ensure that the goals we presumably desire to achieve are accomplished in the most effective ways—ways that do not contribute to normalizing unjust social practices that systematically disadvantage women.

Valuing Mitochondrial Replacement Techniques

Reprogenetic technologies, as we saw in Chapter 7, have the ability to promote, reinforce, challenge, and transform human values. Skepticism about the wisdom of developing and implementing particular technologies can result from these interactions rather than from safety concerns. Importantly, this does not mean that such interactions between human values and technological developments cannot be directed or shaped at all.

But unless these possibilities are recognized, it seems difficult to see how the technologies can be changed in ways that might be found more appropriate.

It seems clear that one of the values advanced by MRTs is that of the importance of a genetic connection between parents and their offspring. As I have indicated, this bond is thought to be essential for many people, and MRTs aim at preserving it. Of course, there is nothing intrinsically problematic with valuing genetic relations. But when this connection is privileged in such a way that it appears morally appropriate to develop risky and expensive technologies despite significant uncertainties about their effects on both the children born through their use and future generations, it is not unreasonable to believe that such privileging has gone a bit too far. That a significant amount of attention has being given to whether children born through MRTs should have access to the identity of the woman who provides the healthy mitochondria only underscores this emphasis on genetic connections.

One might object that all reprogenetic technologies advance the value of a genetic connection between parents and children and that MRTs are not exceptional in this sense. That is certainly true. Indeed, many of our social and institutional practices, not just reprogenetic technologies, privilege, or have the effect of privileging, genetic connections in families. But I hardly need to point out that the fact that other technologies or practices exist that already do this is not a sufficient reason to continue supporting technologies or practices that further this value. As I argued earlier in this chapter, investment in these new technologies has opportunity costs, and other worthy projects—indeed, by any standards, more worthy projects—could be funded in their stead.

The fact that millions of existent children worldwide who are waiting to be adopted could also benefit gives additional reasons to be skeptical of MRTs.[4] Around the world, there are more than 16 million orphans who have lost both parents and are living in orphanages or on the streets without appropriate care. The overwhelming majority of them are in need of parental care. Doubtless, there are reasons other than the privileging of a genetic connection for why the majority of these children are not adopted—they might be sick or "too old," for instance—but undeniably the overvaluing of genetic connections is a very important factor. Furthermore, the very fact that many children get "too old" before they can be adopted is, at least in part, also the result of such overvaluing. Because of institutional barriers, adoptions often involve extensive waiting times and are expensive. But clearly, if as much attention were given to addressing some of those barriers and helping people adopt as is given to developing technological innovations that allow some people to have genetically related offspring, the extensive waiting times and costs could be lessened. It is certainly peculiar, and indeed it is another sign of the inappropriate privileging of genetic connections, that prospective parents might find it easier and more feasible to use reprogenetic technologies than to adopt a child.

One might also argue that it is problematic to expect women who suffer from mitochondrial diseases—or those who are infertile or suffer from other genetic conditions—to shoulder alone that which requires broader social changes. If preference for a genetic connection should not be given such precedence, then this problem of children needing adoption needs to be addressed by all prospective parents and not only to those who are unlucky enough to need reprogenetic technologies. This is correct: Facilitating adoption for all prospective parents is a morally appropriate goal. I agree with others who have argued that

---

4. Clearly, a variety of political, legal, and social factors can make adoption itself a problem, but discussing these issues is beyond the scope of this work.

there is a pro tanto duty to adopt rather than to have genetically related children and that this is a duty that applies to all, not just to those who must use reprogenetics in order to have genetically related offspring (Liao 2006; Rulli 2014). Clearly, however, the development and implementation of new technological interventions that reinforce the value of the genetic connection does nothing to either address broader social changes that would make adoption more feasible or encourage others to adopt.

Equally troubling is that maintaining the genetic connection is thought to be sufficiently important to put others at risk. Perhaps these risks could be justifiably imposed if the presumed benefits were significant and the risks and benefits were fairly distributed. But this is hardly the case as far as MRTs are concerned. Arguably, although the women using these technologies run the risks related to IVF, it is not clear that the children born with the help of MRTs (and their future progeny) will be benefited. Proponents of these technologies contend that such benefits exist because these children and their descendants will be free from mitochondrial disorders. This, however, is questionable because it presupposes that women with the relevant types of mitochondrial disorders who want to become mothers will actually have those children rather than take advantage of existent alternatives (e.g., adoption, egg donation, PGD). It is true that, insofar as women with mtDNA mutations decide to have children, and as long as MRTs are effective, children born through these means, as well as future generations, would benefit.

Furthermore, because these technologies, at least at this point, require the use of other women's eggs, the interest in ensuring a genetic connection is again fulfilled at the cost of putting donor women at risk. It is true that living organ donations always involve risks to donors and that most see these types of donations as morally unproblematic. But usually other living organ donations happen in the context of life-threatening disease.

The value at stake is that of human life rather than that of a genetic connection to offspring. Of course, women who provide the eggs are presumed to be doing so voluntarily. Nonetheless, we have mentioned the lack of studies evaluating the long-term health effects on women who provide eggs or the scarce institutional attention that has been given to developing and enforcing data gathering. Moreover, the increasing phenomenon of cross-border reproductive care calls into question the voluntariness of at least some women's decisions to provide the necessary eggs (Dickenson 2013; Donchin 2010).

Like other reprogenetic technologies, MRTs also embody values about technological fixes. Insofar as the desire for genetically related children is the result of social pressures, the use of medical technologies (with the agreement of the medical profession) to respond to such desire does nothing to address the underlying factors that make the inability to have genetically related offspring a problem in the first place. It is ethically questionable to ignore these aspect of MRTs when assessing these technologies.

Furthermore, as feminist scholars emphasize, science and technology should not serve to reinforce systems of oppression but to challenge such systems (Harding 2008; Kourany 2010; Lacey 2005). Nonetheless, current scientific and technological practices often strengthen a view of science and technology as serving the interests of a few—often those few who can pay for these scientific innovations—rather than also focusing on the needs of the marginalized. As I said earlier, science and technology are public goods and therefore should be conducted in ways that are socially responsive. Many of the diseases that affect the world's poorest people and that constitute a significant burden of disease are neglected (GDB 2015). Indeed, a "10/90 gap" is well documented: Only 10% of worldwide expenditures on health research and development are devoted to the problems that affect primarily the poorest 90% of the world's population

(Kilama 2009; Tomlinson et al. 2014). For many diseases, the problem is not only scarcity of adequate medicines but also a lack of adequate research on strategies other than curative ones (Glasgow and Schrecker 2015; Masters et al. 2014). For example, the enactment of particular social policies might have a more significant effect on reducing the burden of diabetes, obesity, and other chronic conditions than the use of medical interventions. Recall that investments in scientific and technological innovations always have opportunity costs. These costs ought to be taken into account when developing new interventions. However, because technological innovations are more often than not assessed in a vacuum, these costs are routinely ignored.

Conclusion

There is little doubt that MRTs constitute a scientific feat. If effective, they will help some women who are at risk of transmitting mitochondrial disorders to have unaffected and genetically related offspring. This is a good thing. However, this benefit needs to be evaluated against potential alternatives that, as we have seen, might be significantly more cost-effective than MRTs in reducing the burdens of mitochondrial diseases and in allowing women to have genetically related children. In addition, serious concerns exist about potential harms to women undergoing these technologies and to their offspring and future generations. Moreover, because MRTs are qualitatively different from other reprogenetic technologies, known and unknown uncertainties still plague these technologies. The safety questions that still exist make the use of these technologies in human beings at this point questionable, particularly given that MRTs do not address any life-threatening disease and that other alternatives exist to allow women with mitochondrial disorders to become mothers.

Although at least some of those alternatives do not preserve a genetic connection between mother and child, maintaining such a connection arguably should not be a scientific and technological priority. This is the case not because there is something ethically suspect about the desire to have a genetic connection with one's offspring. In a context in which pressing health needs are attended to and unlimited resources are available—a world in which women have control over their bodies and access to contraception as well as food, shelter, education, health care, and day care for their children—the use of scientific and technological resources to preserve women's genetic relations to their children would be unproblematic. But ours is not such world. To ignore the context in which MRTs are developed and implemented is to provide an inadequate assessment of these technologies.

References

Amato, P., M. Tachibana, M. Sparman, and S. Mitalipov. 2014. Three-parent in vitro fertilization: gene replacement for the prevention of inherited mitochondrial diseases. *Fertility and Sterility* 101 (1):31–5.

Barritt, J.A., C.A. Brenner, H.E. Malter, and J. Cohen. 2001. Mitochondria in human offspring derived from ooplasmic transplantation. *Human Reproduction* 16(3):513–6.

Baylis, F. 2013. The ethics of creating children with three genetic parents. *Reproductive Biomedicine Online* 26 (6):531–4.

Begley, C. G., and L. M. Ellis. 2012. Drug development: raise standards for preclinical cancer research. *Nature* 483 (7391):531–3.

Bender, S., L. Flicker, and R. Rhodes. 2007. Access for the terminally ill to experimental medical innovations: a three-pronged threat. *American Journal of Bioethics* 7 (10):3–6.

Bentov, Y., and R. F. Casper. 2013. The aging oocyte: can mitochondrial function be improved? *Fertility and Sterility* 99 (1):18–22.

Braude, P., and Y. Khalaf. 2013. Evidence-based medicine and the role of the private sector in assisted reproduction: a response to Dr

Fishel's commentary 'Evidenced-based medicine and the role of the National Health Service in assisted reproduction.' *Reproductive Biomedicine Online* 27 (5):570–2.

Brighouse, Harry, and Adam Swift. 2014. *Family values: the ethics of parent-child relationships.* Princeton, NJ: Princeton University Press.

Burgstaller, J. P., I. G. Johnston, and J. Poulton. 2015. Mitochondrial DNA disease and developmental implications for reproductive strategies. *Molecular Human Reproduction* 21 (1):11–22.

Calle, A., R. Fernandez-Gonzalez, P. Ramos-Ibeas, R. Laguna-Barraza, S. Perez-Cerezales, P. Bermejo-Alvarez, M. A. Ramirez, and A. Gutierrez-Adan. 2012. Long-term and transgenerational effects of in vitro culture on mouse embryos. *Theriogenology* 77 (4):785–93.

Cil, A. P., and E. Seli. 2013. Current trends and progress in clinical applications of oocyte cryopreservation. *Current Opinion in Obstetrics and Gynecology* 25 (3):247–54.

Cree, L., and P. Loi. 2015. Mitochondrial replacement: from basic research to assisted reproductive technology portfolio tool—technicalities and possible risks. *Molecular Human Reproduction* 21 (1):3–10.

Dickenson, Donna L. 2013. The commercialization of human eggs in mitochondrial replacement research. *The New Bioethics* 19 (1):18–29.

Dobler, R., B. Rogell, F. Budar, and D. K. Dowling. 2014. A meta-analysis of the strength and nature of cytoplasmic genetic effects. *Journal of Evolutionary Biology* 27 (10):2021–34.

Donchin, A. 2010. Reproductive tourism and the quest for global gender justice. *Bioethics* 24 (7):323–32.

Dondorp, W., and G. de Wert. 2011. Innovative reproductive technologies: risks and responsibilities. *Human Reproduction* 26 (7):1604–8.

Dunham-Snary, K. J., and S. W. Ballinger. 2015. Genetics: mitochondrial-nuclear DNA mismatch matters. *Science* 349 (6255):1449–50.

Evers, J. L. 2013. The wobbly evidence base of reproductive medicine. *Reproductive Biomedicine Online* 27 (6):742–6.

GBD 2013 Mortality and Causes of Death Collaborators. 2015. Global, regional, and national age-sex specific all-cause and cause-specific mortality for 240 causes of death, 1990–2013: a systematic analysis for the Global Burden of Disease Study 2013. *Lancet* 385 (9963):117–71.

Glasgow, S., and T. Schrecker. 2015. The double burden of neoliberalism?: noncommunicable disease policies and the global political economy of risk. *Health Place* 34:279–86.

Gorman, G. S., J. P. Grady, Y. Ng, et al. 2015. Mitochondrial donation: how many women could benefit? *New England Journal of Medicine* 372 (9):885–7.

Hackam, D. G., and D. A. Redelmeier. 2006. Translation of research evidence from animals to humans. *JAMA* 296 (14):1731–2.

Harding, Sandra G. 2008. Sciences from below: feminisms, postcolonialities, and modernities. In *Next wave: new directions in women's studies*. Durham, NC: Duke University Press.

Harris, John. 2015a. Germline manipulation and our future worlds. *American Journal of Bioethics* 15 (12):30–4.

———. 2015b. Germline modification and the burden of human existence. *Cambridge Quarterly of Healthcare Ethics* 25 (1):6–18.

(HFE) The human fertilisation and embryology (mitochondrial donation) regulations 2015. 2015. UK Statutory Instrument no. 572. http://www.legislation.gov.uk/uksi/2015/572/contents/made.

(HFEA) Human Fertilisation and Embryology Authority. 2015. *Statement on mitochondrial donation*. http://www.hfea.gov.uk/9606.html.

Jonas, Hans. 1984. *The imperative of responsibility: in search of an ethics for the technological age*. Chicago: University of Chicago Press.

Keehn, J., E. Howell, M. V. Sauer, and R. Klitzman. 2015. How agencies market egg donation on the Internet: a qualitative study. *Journal of Law and Medical Ethics* 43 (3):610–8.

Kilama, Wen L. 2009. The 10/90 gap in sub-Saharan Africa: resolving inequities in health research. *Acta Tropica* 112 (suppl 1):S8–15.

Kohda, T. 2013. Effects of embryonic manipulation and epigenetics. *Journal of Human Genetics* 58 (7):416–20.

Kourany, Janet A. 2010. *Philosophy of science after feminism*. Studies in Feminist Philosophy. New York: Oxford University Press.

Lacey, Hugh. 2005. *Values and objectivity in science*. Lanhm, MD: Rowman and Littlefield.

Leonard, E. W. 2009. Right to experimental treatment: FDA new drug approval, constitutional rights, and the public's health. *Journal of Law and Medical Ethics* 37 (2):269–79.

Liao, S. M. 2006. The right of children to be loved. *Journal of Political Philosophy* 14 (4):420–440.

Lightowlers, R. N., R. W. Taylor, and D. M. Turnbull. 2015. Mutations causing mitochondrial disease: what is new and what challenges remain? *Science* 349 (6255):1494–9.

Masters, W. A., P. Webb, J. K. Griffiths, and R. J. Deckelbaum. 2014. Agriculture, nutrition, and health in global development: typology and metrics for integrated interventions and research. *Annals of the New York Academy of Science* 1331:258–69.

Morrow, E. H., K. Reinhardt, J. N. Wolff, and D. K. Dowling. 2015. Risks inherent to mitochondrial replacement. *EMBO Reports* 16 (5):541–4.

Perel, P., I. Roberts, E. Sena, P. Wheble, C. Briscoe, P. Sandercock, M. Macleod, L. E. Mignini, P. Jayaram, and K. S. Khan. 2007. Comparison of treatment effects between animal experiments and clinical trials: systematic review. *BMJ* 334 (7586):197–200.

Requejo, J. H., and Z. A. Bhutta. 2015. The post-2015 agenda: staying the course in maternal and child survival. *Archives of Disease in Child* 100 Suppl 1:S76–81.

Rubino, P., P. Viganò, A. Luddi, and P. Piomboni. 2016. The ICSI procedure from past to future: a systematic review of the more controversial aspects. *Human Reproduction Update* 22 (2):194–227.

Rulli, Tinal. 2014. The Unique Value of Adoption. In *Family Making: Contemporary Ethical Challenges*, edited by Francoise Baylis and Carolyn McLeod, Oxford University Press, 2014.

Sallevelt, S. C., J. C. Dreesen, M. Drüsedau, et al. 2013. Preimplantation genetic diagnosis in mitochondrial DNA disorders: challenge and success. *Journal of Medical Genetics* 50 (2):125–32.

Say, R. E., R. G. Whittaker, H. E. Turnbull, R. McFarland, R. W. Taylor, and D. M. Turnbull. 2011. Mitochondrial disease in pregnancy: a systematic review. *Obstetric Medicine* 4 (3):90–94.

Sharpley, M. S., C. Marciniak, K. Eckel-Mahan, et al. 2012. Heteroplasmy of mouse mtDNA is genetically unstable and results in altered behavior and cognition. *Cell* 151 (2):333–43.

Smeets, H. J., S. C. Sallevelt, J. C. Dreesen, C. E. de Die-Smulders, and I. F. de Coo. 2015. Preventing the transmission of mitochondrial DNA disorders using prenatal or preimplantation genetic diagnosis. *Annals of the New York Academy of Sciences* 1350:29–36.

Stewart, D. E., B. Rosen, J. Irvine, P. Ritvo, H. Shapiro, J. Murphy, J. Thomas, G. E. Robinson, J. Neuman, and R. Deber. 2001. The disconnect: infertility patients' information and the role they wish to play in decision making. *Medscape Womens Health* 6 (4):1.

Tachibana, Masahito, Paula Amato, Michelle Sparman, et al. 2013. Towards germline gene therapy of inherited mitochondrial diseases. *Nature* 493 (7434):627–31.

Tachibana, Magahito, M. Sparman, H. Sritanaudomchai, H. Ma, L. Clepper, J. Woodward, Y. Li, C. Ramsey, O. Kolotushkina, and S. Mitalipov. 2009. Mitochondrial gene replacement in primate offspring and embryonic stem cells. *Nature* 461 (7262):367–72.

Tatone, C. 2008. Oocyte senescence: a firm link to age-related female subfertility. *Gynecologic Endocrinology* 24 (2):59–63.

Taylor, S., B. Williams, D. Magnus, A. Goenka, and N. Modi. 2015. From MDG to SDG: good news for global child health? *Lancet* 386 (10000):1213–4.

Tomlinson, M., M. H. Bornstein, M. Marlow, and L. Swartz. 2014. Imbalances in the knowledge about infant mental health in rich and poor countries: too little progress in bridging the gap. *Infant Mental Health Journal* 35 (6):624–9.

Uroz, V., and L. Guerra. 2009. Donation of eggs in assisted reproduction and informed consent. *Medical Law* 28 (3):565–75.

Wallace, D. C., and D. Chalkia. 2013. Mitochondrial DNA genetics and the heteroplasmy conundrum in evolution and disease. *Cold Spring Harbor Perspectives in Biology* 5 (11):a021220.

Wang, T., H. Sha, D. Ji, H. L. Zhang, D. Chen, Y. Cao, and J. Zhu. 2014. Polar body genome transfer for preventing the transmission of inherited mitochondrial diseases. *Cell* 157 (7):1591–604.

Wolf, D. P., N. Mitalipov, and S. Mitalipov. 2015. Mitochondrial replacement therapy in reproductive medicine. *Trends in Molecular Medicine* 21 (2):68–76.

Wynne, Brian. 2001. Creating public alienation: expert cultures of risk and ethics on GMOs. *Science as Culture (London)* 10 (4):445–81.

Zhao, Y., P. Brezina, C. C. Hsu, J. Garcia, P. R. Brinsden, and E. Wallach. 2011. In vitro fertilization: four decades of reflections and promises. *Biochimica et Biophysica Acta* 1810 (9):843–52.

INDEX